New Dimensions Books

Larry Dossey

in Conversation with
Michael Toms

Series editor
Hal Zina Bennett, Ph.D.

Published by

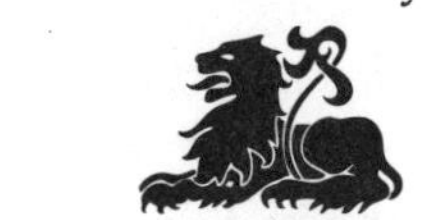

Aslan Publishing
Lower Lake, California
USA

Published by
Aslan Publishing
P.O. Box 108
Lower Lake, CA 95457
(707) 995-1861

For a free catalog of all our titles,
or to order more copies of this book,
please call (800) 275-2606.

Library of Congress Cataloging-in-Publication Data

Dossey, Larry, 1940.
Larry Dossey in conversation with Michael Toms.
p. cm. — (New dimensions books)
ISBN 0-944031-53-6 : $8.95
1. Larry Dossey, 1940—Interviews. 2. Medicine and psychology. 3. Mind and body. 4. Medicine, Psychosomatic. 5. Holistic medicine. I. Toms, Michael. II. Title. III. Series.
R726.5.D67 1994
610′.1—dc20 94-22645
CIP

Cover photo by Athi-Mara
Cover design by Channing Rudd
Printed in USA

10 9 8 7 6 5 4 3 2 1

Quotes About Michael Toms

". . . one of the best interviewers who has ever worked the American airwaves, radio or TV."

—Robert Fuller
Physicist, educator, past president of Oberlin College, and active citizen diplomat

"Someone with whom I have cruised some important realms of the cosmic ocean and in doing so have developed ever increasing confidence in his intuitive navigation."

—R. Buckminster Fuller (1895–1983)
Inventor of the geodesic dome, designer, philosopher, and creator of the World Game

". . . Bill Moyers and Michael Toms are alike: two of the most creative interviewers it has been my good fortune to work with."

—Joseph Campbell (1904–1987)
Mythologist and author of *Hero with a Thousand Faces, The Masks of God, Myths to Live By,* and *The Mythic Image*

Table of Contents

Series Introduction

Through a cooperative arrangement between New Dimensions Radio and Aslan Publishing, we are pleased to present these highly readable introductions to some of the finest and most influential minds of our times. This series of books grew out of interviews broadcast by New Dimensions Radio and conducted by Michael Toms, who is arguably the most articulate, insightful and well-read radio personality of our times.

A non-profit educational organization, New Dimensions Radio has dedicated its efforts, for over twenty years, to fostering communication about personal and social transformation through regular weekly interviews with some of the world's most prominent men and women in science, religion, psychology, philosophy, ecology, and virtually every discipline.

In 1973, Michael and Justine Toms were inspired by a comment made by Charles Tart, a renowned researcher in altered states of consciousness. Tart had remarked that we were "in the midst of the most dramatic shift in human consciousness in the history of the planet—and nobody is paying attention." Convinced that Tart was right, and that the mass media were particularly resistant to what was happening, Michael and Justine stepped boldly forward and launched New Dimensions Radio, originally through KQED-FM in San Francisco. Michael has served as principal host and executive producer during all that time, with Justine acting as program and series director.

Today, New Dimensions Radio boasts a broadcast network of more than two-hundred stations throughout the United States and abroad. These programs are carried worldwide through short-wave radio and via satellite on the Armed Forces Radio Network. Together, Michael and Justine have pioneered a new style of "compassionate journalism," which fosters open dialogue and clear communication intended to empower listeners. Their weekly listenership has now reached more than three-million worldwide, while the roster of their interviewees includes Nobel Prize physicists, holistic physicians, artists, healers, world renowned spiritual leaders, and notables such as Buckminster Fuller, Maya Angelou, Jean Houston, Joseph Campbell, and the Dalai Lama.

Our goal in this series is to offer books that extend Michael and Justine Toms's ambitious efforts from the airwaves to the printed page, probing the minds of our country's leading thinkers, recording their thoughts and feelings as well as the essence of their own works. In these books, we feel that we have been able to capture more than the intellectual side of the great minds of our generation; in addition, we've been able to catch glimpses of these great minds as people, touched by those events of everyday life that we all know so well. These are books that allow us to share how these outstanding minds incorporate their ideas into their own daily life processes.

By virtue of the more informal interviews, which are the basis of these books, we get to know the more human side of the interviewees, their doubts, fears, and private aspirations. These candid insights are only rarely found in more formal books and lectures. They are important because they help us bring down to earth works that we might otherwise think are beyond our own capacities. In this way, the great works of our time become much more accessible, much more user-friendly, and applicable in our own lives.

At the time the publisher came to me with the idea for this series, I had been an avid New Dimensions Radio listener almost since its inception. I had even enjoyed the honor of being interviewed by the Tomses over the years, talking about my own books or books I had co-authored. But most of all, the interviews I heard on this series were often my introduction to the real giants at the cutting edge of science, psychology, the social sciences, spirituality, the arts and self-development.

From the beginning, we have all been excited by the opportunity to present in this highly readable form ideas that are helping to make this a better world. It is our hope that whether you are reading these ideas for the first time, or have picked up this book to refresh your memory of a lecture, book or workshop that previously acquainted you with these authors' works, that you will be moved as profoundly as we have been by their efforts.

Throughout our publishing program, we continue to dedicate ourselves to bringing you the works of men and women who are amongst the most creative, thought-provoking, and controversial on this planet. We hope you will look for other books in this continuing series, since together they present the ideas that are truly changing the world for the better.

—Hal Zina Bennett, Ph.D.

Introduction

Did you ever wonder about your mind? It's paradoxical, isn't it? We have to use the mind to explore the mind, a task which might seem somewhat akin to pulling ourselves up by our own bootstraps. However, there is sufficient evidence to suggest that the mind is non local—in other words, not confined to the cortex or even to the physical body. Rather, it may be that our minds extend far beyond the boundaries of physical limitations, into a larger, even infinite realm. It is perhaps this aspect of the mind that has led to the great breakthroughs in modern physics in recent years, wherein researchers seem to have gained the ability to use the mind to stand outside and observe the mind. And it is out of this new science that Larry Dossey, M.D., has begun to develop the revolutionary view of health and healing that is examined in this book.

Larry Dossey, M.D., has applied the insights of quantum physics to the healing process, telling how we can transform our health and our lives through releasing our limitations of mind. he believes that our attitudes, perceptions, the way we think the world works, and how we interpret what happens around us directly affects our health.

An internal medicine specialist, Larry has always been intrigued by his patients who experienced "miracle cures"—recoveries that couldn't be explained by clinical medicine. A leading advocate of mind-body medicine, he explores the reasons for such recoveries, discovering that at least some of the answers can be found in the meaning people attribute to their lives and their illnesses.

According to Dr. Dossey, modern medical science threw out concepts like health, illness, and wellness when they rejected soul, mind and consciousness. He tells us that most of modern medicine teaches that illness is just our molecules and atoms gone awry and that how we perceive and experience our lives plays no part in health and illness. if this is true, Dr. Dossey asks, why is job dissatisfaction the most important contributing factor in first heart attacks, overriding almost every other medical risk? Why do we attribute the wish *to die* to patients who feel trapped in their lives, and the *will to live* to those who survive against all odds? And how is it that hearts can actually break from the grief of losing a loved one?

In this dialogue with Larry Dossey, we explore the issues of health and the human mind. Larry refers time and time again to the possibility that each of us can constructively alter what we view as meaningful in our lives and what we might view in the face of illness. His ideas lead the way to a new era in medicine, literally a new medical age. His rich and varied clinical experience, combined with his extensive knowledge of modern science, provides the basis for urging modern medicine forward, into the realms of the healing powers of the body-mind and even the body-soul.

Dr. Dossey suggests that the dichotomy between allopatric medicine and more holistic approaches to health and healing are beginning to be resolved as we see new ways to approach science. He sees that we are moving toward a balance between allopatric medicine, as it is now practiced, and the new views of our world that are offered by that more precise science, modern physics. By changing our outmoded views of mind and matter, and their relationship to the universe, the healing arts can once more regain stature as caring and humane, even while sharing a firm foundation of scientific discipline.

The author of numerous articles and five highly acclaimed books on mind-body health, Dr. Dossey has lectured throughout the world on how physical health and spiritual development are synergistic. His ideas are practical and easy to follow, with an abundance of useful information for medical practitioners and lay people alike. Perhaps the most interesting and awesome aspect of Dr. Dossey's message is that virtually everything he says is supported by empirical data.

In this book, Dr. Dossey gives us a glimpse of how he sees modern medicine evolving, revealing powerful new attitudes of what true health is all about.

—Michael Toms
Ukiah, California

Section One

The Search for Meaning—
Medicine of the Future

MICHAEL: *There comes a time for most of us when we consciously seek to bring a sense of meaning into our lives, to be engaged in activities and purposes that we feel are truly meaningful. But Larry Dossey takes this quest to new levels. He tells us that how we perceive, feel, and think relates directly to our overall health. Modern medical science has not yet accepted the link between meaning and health, illness and wellness. However, there are a few pioneering physicians—and Larry is clearly at the head of the pack—who are leading the way toward a new vision of meaning into the healing process.*

Larry, I would like to begin this interview by asking you to tell us a story. It is one you have previously shared with me about screwworms, *and it is important because it deeply influenced you at an early age, and led to your present interests and research.*

LARRY: I grew up on a sharecropper cotton farm in the middle of the state of Texas; a few acres of cotton, corn, and a few cows. Back in those days there was a pestilence that really was terrible for these farmers, although it's been eradicated now. Screwworms were a tremendous problem. Flies would lay their eggs in an open cut or wound and the worms would develop and bore into the flesh and frequently kill the animal. The recommended treatments were to cauterize and scrape out the wound and to pour toxic chemicals into it to kill any more eggs and worms. This just didn't work in one particular calf my father was treating. And so one day he took me with him to go get a "curandera," a Mexican woman who could talk out the worms. She came and talked to the worms, in solitude. The worms left, almost immediately, before my very eyes. I asked my father how this was possible. And he said to me that Maria knows what this disease means. She has reasoned with the worms, she told them that this calf had been willful and had tried to jump a fence, and so cut himself on the barbed wire. She told the calf to rethink that kind of behavior, and she told the worms if they stayed there they would kill the calf and they and the calf would all die. So she struck these bargains with the calf and the worms and they all understood the meaning of the problem.

This experience always stayed with me. I was never able to get it out of my mind. When I went to medical school all this was swept aside. Physicians are told, even today, that disease has no meaning. It's just a matter of what your atoms and molecules and organs happen to be doing. But later, after going into the practice of medicine, the issue of meaning once again reasserted itself for me. I found that I could not understand the diseases my patients were getting without bringing meaning into the equation. So, although I tried to forget the impact of meaning, I couldn't, and I began exploring how meanings affect the body and what they have to do with any given illness.

You had the experience in medical school of having migraine headaches. In fact you had them as a teenager, I seem to recall, and it carried into medical school. You started worrying about how this might affect your future medical practice. Can you tell us about that?

I recall my first migraine headache when I was about age fourteen. These were sensational headaches, with partial blindness, nausea, vomiting and feeling wiped out for twenty four hours. Frankly, I lied on my medical school admission form; I did not report this as a medical problem. During the stress of medical school the headaches simply got a lot worse. I was worried that I would be in surgery or in a resuscitation attempt and would suffer an episode of blindness. I was afraid I really might kill someone. So this took on ethical dimensions for me and I even went to my faculty advisor and told him that I was going to drop out of medical school. He persuaded me not to do that.

None of the therapies that medicine had to offer worked until I discovered, years later, biofeedback and learning to control aspects of my own physiology. That was like a wake up call for me. It was an undeniable connection between my mind and my body and it forced me to look at the meaning of those headaches in my own life. I was a very driven person; I did nearly everything on automatic pilot. This was not a very satisfying way to go through life and I was paying the price for it. So, the meaning of that personal illness was very graphic in my mind and was very influential, basically changing my life and my focus and my way of seeing the importance of meaning and illness. I had to change the way I approached my work, and my life, or the headaches were just going to get worse and worse.

In Meaning and Medicine *you spoke of particular stresses associated with medical school, and how they may actually set people up for certain diseases, particularly cancer…*

That's exactly right. One of the great clinical studies of modern medical research was done by a woman named Caroline Thomas at Johns Hopkins Medical School. She did psychological testing for twenty-three years on every medical student who came through the doors at that school. She followed these students for decades and correlated patterns in their psychological profiles with the diseases they eventually developed and died from. In cancer there were stunning, almost chilling, correlations between the disease and the psychological profile. Those students who could not express emotion, who kept things bottled up, who couldn't get it out, had the strongest tendency to develop cancer and die from it.

For me Dr. Thomas's studies are particularly telling because they suggest that medical schools may be selecting students with what ultimately amounts to very unhealthy coping styles, or that the school is actually grooming them, or both. At the very least we can say that the way medical schools are run today support people in lifestyles which are very unhealthy and which possibly contribute to their eventual diseases.

The psychological profile in question is one that emphasizes the head, along with the denial of emotion. The coping style is to keep things bottled up, like saying, "Boy, that hurts so much! Can you give me a little bit more of that?" That's the kind of crazy, psychological style that is guaranteed to get you ahead in medical school. This says something very worrisome about education, not just in medical school but in other professional schools as well. What are we doing to our students when we encourage that kind of psychological coping style? This way of being may get you ahead in those schools, but apparently it also sets you up as a prime candidate for cancer.

So, if what you're saying is true, aren't you also suggesting that doctors are being trained not to get involved with their patients at an emotional level? Getting close will only cause problems. Yet, you're also saying that physicians should *be involved—that this involvement is a necessary aspect of healing—and, if we extend this viewpoint, is a necessary part of physicians themselves staying healthy and having a healthy impact on their patients.*

Precisely. Let the feelings come out. Allow oneself to be compassionate. Allow oneself to care. Allow oneself to cry if necessary. It's just unfortunate that this myth of the detached, cold, remote physician has become such a dominant force in medicine. Physicians pride themselves on being remote, on not being personally touched by the suffering they witness. And the price we all pay is not just in the inhumane regard for the patient but in the negative health outcomes for the doctors themselves. It's as if we have planted a powerful seed of disease right in the middle of the very system we have developed for treating illness.

In all your books, you've explored the spiritual underpinnings of health. But you addressed this issue most directly in your book Recovering the Soul. *I am wondering, what exactly is the relationship between "recovering the soul" and what you describe as "meaning?"*

Before I answer that, Michael, I want to make a personal comment here. I guess all writers have a favorite book, and *Recovering the Soul* comes close to being that for me. That book is all about meaning. The most wretched, horrible aspect of existence for most of us is this idea that when we die, it's all over. That is the most powerful negative meaning anyone can live with. That book was an attempt to address this issue and restore the idea of the soul, the belief that something survives the death of brain and body. It's the most powerful meaning we can have—that in essence we are immortal, eternal, and omnipresent. For me, bringing that kind of meaning back into people's lives is one of the most therapeutic insights a physician can offer.

You make a point in that book that it is very difficult in medicine to get people to recognize the existence of anything that isn't visible. Just as the soul is invisible—you can't measure it or weigh it—meaning is also invisible. It presumably can't be measured, weighed, or seen. You can't scientifically quantify it. So what cannot be measured or seen, that is, what is invisible in our lives, tends to be excluded from medicine, dismissed as irrelevant or even nonexistent.

Right. We have literally been taught that if something is not measurable we're not to concern ourselves with it. So, we're in trouble where meaning and the soul are concerned.

We can't plug into a human body and take a direct reading that might indicate their presence.

You know, it's very odd that in light of what modern science has learned anyone in our society would still measure reality on the basis of something being visible or invisible. That whole notion is obsolete—it ought to go by the wayside. If you look at what happens in the most accurate sciences—in quantum mechanics, subatomic physics and so on — we suddenly discover that they are often working completely with invisible entities. No one has ever held an electron in their hands or seen it with their eyes! Scientists look for the indirect impact of these phenomena on the world. They are literally saying we know these things exist not because they saw them with their own eyes but because what they observe could not be true unless these invisible entities had been there. Ken Wilbur says that the soul, the spirit, behaves in much the same way. It leaves its tracks in the world and it is perfectly legitimate, even in scientific terms, to point to these tracks as evidence for the existence of soul and spirit.

Recovering the Soul was my effort to say, look, there are an awful lot of tracks out there, offering reasonable, empirical evidence that there is an aspect of our psyche that cannot be identified in terms of specific points in space and time. There are tracks suggesting that the soul is omnipresent and infinite, outside time and space, immortal and eternal. I believe we are at a sensational turning point in human history, where for the first time we have demonstrated very strong empirical evidence for the existence of something that resembles the soul. That's what this book was designed to show, to explore.

As you speak, I am thinking that meaning itself, though invisible, has an impact not just on our intellectual lives but also on our physical lives, on our bodies. You seem to be suggesting that whenever there is the presence of an illness we should perhaps be looking for how it is an expression of a meaning. Maybe we'll discover that the illness is the track, as you put it, of the meaning this person has held in his or her life.

Yes. We plow our meanings into our bodies, with very definite results. These results may be negative or they may be positive but they will clearly have an impact on our bodies. As an example let's take the commonest killer in our culture today—heart disease. Heart disease kills more people than all other diseases combined. And yet, we have come to think of this disease not in terms of meaning or consciousness so much as in terms of the so-called *major risk factors:* cholesterol, smoking, high blood pressure, diabetes.

However, as it turns out, in the United States, most people under the age of fifty, as a man named Jenkins showed in 1971, have none of these major risk factors when they suffer their first heart attack. This suggests that something has been left out of the heart attack profile. But what is it? The further we explore this issue, the stranger it gets. For example, we discover that more heart attacks occur in this country on Monday than on any other day of the week, and they cluster from 8:00 to 9:00 in the morning. This is the so called "Black Monday Syndrome," which is a chapter in my book *Meaning and Medicine.*

If you can't predict the occurrence of heart disease in the majority of cases, by looking at what medicine has identified as the major risk factors, what do you look at? A study done in the state of Massachusetts in the early seventies showed that if you want to predict who is going to have their first heart attack under the age of fifty, the best predictor is their level of job dissatisfaction. Now, what this is telling us is that *meaning* enters the body and literally becomes a life-and-death matter.

Why is job dissatisfaction so important? What does a job mean to us? What does your job conjure in your mind? What does it symbolize? Stand for? What does it represent? What is the meaning of work in your life? This meaning is either negative or positive and it's plowed into the body— that's what we must look at if we are to begin to understand illness and health.

As far as we know, human beings are the only species on the face of the earth who manage to die more frequently on a particular day of the week. We are also the only species, we believe, who finds meaning in things. And so, I believe that we can't expect to understand the origin of the commonest things that kill us if we don't bring meaning into the equation.

So, in the most simplistic terms, if you don't like your job, you better find another one you do like for the sake of your health.

That's what it comes down to. I had one patient offer an alternate solution, however. She suggested that instead of going in on Mondays, she go in on Tuesdays. But of course, if we did that we would soon be talking about the "Black Tuesday Syndrome."

We should be looking at meaning as seriously as we look at cholesterol levels or blood pressure, diet, exercise, and even relaxation for stress reduction. It may not be fashionable to do so but the data is out there to support the fact that meaning may be one of the most important disease factors in our lives. For me, as a physician, not to ask a patient about meaning in his or her life, say when they come in for an annual checkup, would be the equivalent of saying, "oops, I forgot to do the physical or to check your blood pressure." It's probably more unforgivable not to inquire about the meaning of work than it would be to forget these other factors.

I think it's interesting that Freud, just before he died, made a statement about the two most important things in life: love and work. It certainly appears that the meaning of work is a powerful predictor of life and death factors.

As you were speaking, I was reminded of an old homily that goes something like, "Nobody on their deathbed ever said they wish they had spent more time at the office."

Yes. That's it. There was a fascinating study from Yale Medical School, early in 1991, conducted by two researchers named Kasl and Idler. The question they wanted to address was this: If we are going to predict who's going to be alive at the end of a decade, what's the best thing to look at? Doctors would say, well, you ought to look at the family history; do they have any genetic diseases? Others would say, check what the physical exam shows or what the lab tests turn up, and all that kind of thing. However, Kasl and Idler found that the single best predictor of longevity was the answer that people gave to a simple question: "What do you think about your health?" If people said my health is excellent, they had only a one-seventh risk of dying over the next decade, compared to a person who said, "I think my health is lousy," or

"I'm really worried about it." This was true even when the people who said their health was bad had recently received a normal physical exam. And it was true even when the people who said their health was excellent had terrible physical exams. In this study, which looked at almost 3,000 subjects, it was clear that people had a way of living out their meanings. Again, there was evidence that we channel whatever meaning we hold within our consciousness right into the body.

Larry, there was a story you related in Meaning and Medicine *about a woman patient whose physician was treating her for heart disease and...well, you're nodding...would you finish that story?*

I'm glad you reminded me. This woman had a heart condition and was actually doing quite well. She had been followed at this cardiac clinic, at this famous medical school, and her physician was one of the most famous cardiologists in the United States. She revered this man. She would hang on his every word. At the time, she was working as a librarian and her heart disease was doing very well.

One day she came in for a routine check. The doctor that she so revered came in, in a big hurry, put his stethoscope to her chest, and without speaking to her turned to the resident physician who happened to be with him and simply said: "T.S." The woman interpreted this to mean "terminal situation." She took it to me she was dying. Actually T.S. meant *tricuspid stenosis,* which refers to one of the valves being stuck, and so on, which happened to be the origin of this woman's heart problem.

Before the hour was out this woman had begun to live out what she interpreted to be a pronouncement of doom. She went into congestive heart failure, developed pulmonary edema, in which her lungs filled with fluid, was admitted to the hospital and within hours was dead.

... even though she learned before she died that nobody had ever actually considered her condition terminal.

Right. That's right. She blocked out that information and lived out the negative meaning.

Now, before we go much further with this, it should be pointed out that positive meanings can have as dramatic impacts on our health as the negative ones. Let me give you an example of how this might work. Dr. David Speigel was a psychiatrist who was an archenemy of this idea that emotions and meanings have anything to do with the course of cancer. He set out over ten years ago to do a study that would once and for all prove that meanings and emotions didn't matter. He brought about 90 women together who had metastatic breast cancer and all of these women were treated conventionally with surgery, chemotherapy, radiation and so on. He taught half of these women some self-hypnosis techniques and importantly brought them together to share their feelings in a group therapy session once a week for a year. These women talked about what it was like, what it means to have metastatic breast cancer, what it means to have chemotherapy and basically be in this situation. Well, when Speigel looked at the survival data ten years later, he was shocked. Mind you, he was a skeptic about this stuff. He found that those women who came together once a week to share their meanings had a doubled life span following their diagnosis compared to those women who just had chemotherapy, radiation and surgery. This is a way in which meaning can be used positively. You see, meaning can kill. That's what we learn from the woman who interpreted tricuspid stenosis to mean "terminal situation." But meaning can also be used as a therapy. Meaning can preserve life. It can heal. That's the wonderful upbeat side of this.

I believe that in the future we will make room in medicine for something we might call "Meaning Therapy." There are a lot of Meaning Therapies out there now that really do focus on manipulation of meaning but we just don't call them that. Dr. Dean Ornish, for example, is a well-known cardiologist who did one of the great meaning studies of the past decade. He took a group of men who were washed up with coronary artery disease and taught them to rearrange their meanings. These men—many had angina at rest, heart pain on doing nothing—which is a terrible prognostic indicator in heart disease.

Several of these men had already had one, two and three by-pass operations. There was nothing that conventional medicine could offer a lot of these people. Dr. Ornish put them on a stringent low-fat diet, taught them some yoga exercises, some meditation and importantly brought them together for group therapy one session a week so that they could explore the meaning of their disease. They asked questions such as, "What does it mean to have this disease? What does it mean to know that you're not going to be able to return to work? What does it mean to know that you are just sitting around waiting for the big one to happen?"

At the end of one year Ornish restudied these men, using sophisticated cardiac catheterization techniques, and these people who came together and shared their feelings and explored their meanings actually had a reversal of their physical conditions. There was a reduction in the size of the coronary lesions, which are made up of cholesterol, placque and scar tissue. It has been said in American medicine as long as I can remember, that once you've got these lesions they are there until you die. You can by-pass them or do something else to try to surgically fix them but they are not going to go away. Ornish showed that if you fix your meanings you can reverse heart disease. He was also able to show, from other previous studies, that if you just do the diet that's not enough. If you just do the stress management, the relaxation, the meditation and yoga, that's not enough either. If you do the meditation, the yoga and the diet, that won't reverse the lesions. What you have to do to reverse the heart disease is do all these and explore the meanings at a very deep level.

Meaning Therapy, I believe, is an extremely powerful form of intervention and we'll be seeing more of it in the years ahead.

In your books, you bring up the subject of voodoo. Maybe you could tell us how this relates to the new meaning therapies?

Well, voodoo is a very legitimate phenomenon. Most of us think that it is not to be taken seriously because it is all just a lot of superstition and old wive's tales. But actually it has been studied scientifically and shown to be extremely important in terms of our understanding the relationships between meaning and health. The bottom line is that the person who is voodoo-hexed lives out the meaning of the curse. He cooperates with it, goes along with it and ultimately manifests the prediction that he or she is going to die.

We know quite a bit about the psychophysiology of voodoo. We know that there are pathways between the brain and the heart and the immune system that really impact dramatically on health. Certain emotions, or meanings, greatly depress the immune system and other aspects of the body's homeostatic processes. Some of the deadliest emotions in this respect are guilt and shame. Now, what happens in voodoo is that the person is tremendously shamed. Negative, guilt-ridden shamefulness messages are imparted to the victim. And the person who believes in that tradition, who has been raised with it, will experience this psychophysiological process and will die from it.

It is interesting to look at our own culture and ask, do we have any modern corollaries with this voodoo hex-type situation, where shame and guilt impact the body and cause illness or death? I think the answer is an unequivocal *yes.* One such corollary I might mention is the way we force early retirement on people who really value their work. If a person's self-esteem is really tied up with their work, their way of thinking about who they are and what their lives are about, these people are at high risk. They feel discounted and humiliated by early retirement, as if they are being told that they are no longer useful, no longer valid or viable members of society. They are, in a sense, hexed by the same society they have been serving all their lives. We know that such people, forced to retire in shame, feel that their lives are no longer meaningful, and they soon get sick and die.

How many people like this die within their first year of retirement?

Well, I don't have the numbers at my fingertips but the figures are incredibly high. As a matter of fact, for certain men whose identity is really tied up with their jobs, forced early retirement is tantamount to a death sentence. The mortality rate is really awesome with this group. They see their whole lives as over—and, of course, that's exactly what happens. Their lives seem to them to have lost all meaning. They die.

Another way we hex people, performing the voodoo rites of our own culture, is by imparting guilt and shame when we involuntarily commit people to nursing homes. This is a way of saying you're no longer important to us. You're no longer worthwhile. We are ostracizing you, banishing you from participating in mainstream culture. You are now set aside. This is precisely the dynamic that goes on in primitive cultures in the voodoo-hex situation. All too frequently, when they are set aside in nursing homes and treated differently, people take on guilt and shame and die precipitously.

There have been studies done with people in nursing homes where they are given certain jobs to do, such as taking care of a potted plant or designing their own menus, in an effort to restore their sense of worthiness and self-esteem. It's interesting that in these situations, even little acts such as these can help restore self-esteem, and can greatly reduce mortality rates in this group. Just giving someone a little bit to do can make such an enormous difference with them.

There are many fascinating stories you tell about the power of voodoo, and one that sticks in my mind concerns this young man who was raised in a culture where it was taboo to eat chicken. He was given chicken to eat and told that it was something else, and suffered no ill effects until much later when he…but maybe you should tell the story.

Yes, yes. This is a story recorded by one of the early Spanish explorers from his experiences in the Congo in the 1500's. The story goes that there was a young man from a culture that was forbidden to eat chicken. However, one night he was dining with a person from another tribe who served him chicken but told him it was the meat of some other animal. There was no malice intended and, of course, nothing happened. The young man who had grown up believing one should never eat chicken went on his way and was perfectly healthy and happy. Then, two years later, he ran into the friend who'd given him the meal of chicken and after some exchange of news they started talking about their previous meeting and their meal together. Somehow it came out that the meat they had eaten that day was chicken. The man for whom this was considered taboo immediately viewed himself as hexed, in spite of the fact that two years had passed without any bad effects. Within twenty-four hours he was dead.

There is another aspect to the affects of meaning on health and illness, however, and this one has to do with our interpretations of what role a disease plays in our lives. This is particularly prevalent with New Agers. Let's say someone has lung cancer, and they've always been a smoker. There are several levels to explore here if you want to get at the meaning of disease in this case. On the most superficial level the disease means that the person shouldn't have smoked. The person had a hand in causing this because of their habit of smoking. I don't know very many people who would argue that. Smoking does contribute to lung cancer, emphysema, and heart disease. So that's one level of meaning with lung cancer. Does it mean anything deeper than that? Could the disease also reflect certain attitudes and emotions, a certain psychological profile, or that you somehow bring a disease into your life through some need in your life? There are certainly a lot people who believe that the answer to this question is yes.

Just recently a woman wrote me and said she'd broken her ankle and she was convinced it was because she was so hesitant to step forward in life. A seventy-year-old woman with severe osteoporosis, and a profound bowing of her upper spine, a humpback, said she knew this had happened because she had trouble bearing her burdens. But are these the real meanings, and did those meanings contribute to those diseases? I'm not sure it's that simplistic.

There are books out there which provide one column listing the disease, and a corresponding column naming the presumed negative feeling state or attitude that caused that disease. In a third column you've got the remedy, the preferred mental state to reverse the disease. All very neat and tidy, a literal readout of disease and meaning. Presumably, it is based on the belief that we create our own illnesses, and just as we create them we can reverse the process and create health.

I go back and forth about all this and I don't think we've got a good handle on it. Let me tell you one reason why. There are not a lot of things that psychiatrists agree about today, but the thing they do agree on is that at least 90 percent of our psychological life is spent in non-awareness. Ninety percent of our psychological life is probably unconscious. Wouldn't this mean that there is about a 10 percent chance that we are conscious of creating our disease but that there is a 90 percent chance that we do so unconsciously, if we do it at all?

If we say that we caused an illness, we are contradicting what most psychiatrists observe in their practices—that most of our behavior is unconscious. If we say we caused our illness mentally, but we weren't aware of doing it, we are really getting into a gray area. What does it mean to say I caused the disease if I wasn't conscious of doing so? We need to be very careful here.

I believe there's some real wisdom in that bumper sticker that was so popular a couple years ago, the one that said: "Shit happens." I think it does happen. And I think that sometimes disease can occur without any cooperation from us, without any creation from us. Sometimes, because it comes from the unconscious, it's impossible to say I caused it. There is also the problem that the unconscious speaks in symbols, never in a rational, linear fashion, and these symbols can be so opaque that even when we are aware that a symbol is involved we still have difficulty understanding its meaning.

I must say that the more I think about the meaning of specific illnesses the more difficult it is for me to accept simplistic readout formulas for what any particular disease *means.* I think the real meaning is often a great mystery and I am very skeptical about trivializations in this area. I think we should always expect to struggle to understand the meaning of any given illness but I also believe that we are limited in our ability to explore the depths of the unconscious where we might find our answers.

I think there is a point with many illnesses when we have to say, "I believe there is a meaning here but I just can't get my hands on it." Sometimes the meanings we seek will bubble to the surface or otherwise announce themselves unexpectedly to us. Sometimes we simply have to wait with openness and try to achieve certain states of awareness that allow the meaning to speak to us instead of us trying to impose our own private and personal meanings on the disease.

I was thinking about that much-overused phrase, that we each create our own reality. Within that framework, it is presumed that if you have cancer, you created it. But in point of fact you are saying we may not have created it at all, at least not consciously, and maybe not even unconsciously. It's very mysterious—we don't really know.

That word "mystery" is key. I think that a quick look at the health histories of some of the God-realized saints and mystics could tell us a lot about the meaning of illness. Frequently their health is wretched. Three of the holiest men I know in this century died of cancer—Krishnamurti died of cancer of the pancreas; Suzuki Roshi, who brought Zen to the

San Francisco Bay Area from Japan, died of cancer of the liver; and the most beloved saint in modern India, Ramana Maharshi, died a horrible death of cancer of the stomach. What does disease mean in their case? Did they create it? If we say yes—and we can say yes, I suppose—what are we actually saying? We're saying that these God-realized people, these Olympic-class spiritual achievers, had no power over their illness and apparently were not able to stop whatever they were doing that was creating it. If they can't make it come out okay, at least in terms of our present assumptions about disease, then what about our own limitations?

I think that Ramana Maharshi's experience in his last days is very instructive here. Dying of cancer, he would awaken in the middle of the night with horrible pain. He would scream out so that his devotees could not sleep, and this created enormous self-doubt in them, as you might imagine. "Why are we studying with this dying man who is supposed to teach us wisdom and how to be healthy?" they would ask each other.

Toward morning, as the cancer pain eased, as it typically does, Maharshi would gather his devotees around him and use this as a teaching opportunity. He would tell them, "Look, the problem is that you identify me with my body. I do not identify myself with my body." So his meaning of the disease was entirely different for him than it was for them. What was his view of the disease, in terms of his having created it or not? We don't know for certain, but what is certain is that we need to be very careful in assigning quick or easy meanings to disease.

I think of Ramakrishna, in the 19th century, who also died of cancer. His disciples asked him why he didn't heal himself. He said: "Well, why should I spend energy on that?" He didn't identify himself with his body and wanted his disciples to learn from this. But I have to ask, isn't there a danger there, too, in that if we dissociate from our bodies, we're not dealing with our existence here on Earth?

Well, in the case of these men, I don't think we're looking at classic dissociation, where a person just says, whatever happens to my body just happens. Nor are we looking at the opposite extreme of this, what Jung called inflation of the ego, or what the ancient Greeks called arrogance, the notion that I can control every single aspect of my life. These are the extremes. Somewhere in between is a proper balance. I think one of the toughest jobs on the spiritual path is to try to find that balance. I suspect it may be different for different people.

But I don't think we can ignore the fact, in the examples that you give, that particularly in Hinduism, with which all four of the people we've discussed are associated, there is this constant drive to leave the body, to go beyond it.

Your point is well-taken, of course. But we need not limit ourselves to examples from the east. In the West, out of the Christian tradition, we've seen other examples of God-realized saints and mystics who succumbed to terrible diseases and expressed similar insights about their life meaning.

One of the most famous cases in the west was that of Bernadette who saw the vision at Lourdes where all the miracles have happened. When Bernadette needed a miracle she didn't get one. She developed bone cancer and died a very painful death at the ripe age of 35. So, this is not just an eastern phenomenon of the God-realized saints and mystics not having a healing when it looks like they need it. Sri Aurobindo was another example. He took a wrong step once and sprained his knee. A devotee who was following him around said, "Boy, this is crazy!" He said, "Master you can see the future,"—and it's true, Aurobindo was famous for being clairvoyant—"why could you not avoid that misstep? You certainly could see that it was coming." And Aurobindo said, "As long as I have a body that body will be subject to the same laws that govern all physical bodies." For him there was no contradiction to having a physical problem and being spiritually mature, while for most of us this contradiction gives us a lot of trouble.

Manly Hall once said he was always running into people in this culture who kept getting God mixed up with vitamins. His point was that we relate to God as a kind of remedy for our ills, in the same way that we might take a vitamin pill or a yoga class or go to a doctor for a certain medication or surgery. He commented that this seems to be the way we do things in the west. We think that we create our realities to such a degree that if we are just spiritual enough, get the right exercise and eat healthy foods we should be able to ward off all physical problems. I just don't think it's that simple.

Often, I think, when we have a problem, particularly an illness, we think we have to do something. And many times that's not the case at all, is it? (Larry nods his head yes.) *Many times it's a matter of just relaxing into the process. You had a section in your book* Meaning and Medicine *about the place of emptiness…*

It seems very difficult for westerners to do nothing and just *be*. Yet, enormously powerful healings can come out of not doing, *that is, simply being and finding that place of emptiness and nothingness and settling into it.*

There's a wonderful story about this that came out of one of the great adventures of all time, the International Trans-Antarctic Expedition. Six men from different countries walked 3,741 miles across Antarctica. It took them nine months. They endured two months of storms, temperatures as low as minus 70 degrees, and so on. Two days before they were to complete this journey disaster struck. They found themselves in a white-out condition in a terrible blizzard.

One of the people on the team was a Japanese man by the name of Keizo Funatsu, who was an expert with sled dogs. At about four-o'clock he went out to feed the huskies and didn't come back. He got lost in the blizzard. He knew that the way these things usually turn out is that you meander a little bit here, a little bit there, and pretty soon you can't find your way back to the tent. Later, you're found dead, frozen solid by the next morning. Keizo decided that he didn't want to run that risk, so instead of doing something he decided to do as little as he could do in that situation. He just kicked a trench in the snow and laid down in it.

He recorded in his diary profound states of feeling that he experienced in those thirteen hours that he lay buried in the snow. He was doing nothing. You know, when you are buried alive, this is about as profound a state of emptiness and doing nothing as anyone can experience. Thirteen hours later, he heard his teammates calling his name, though they were certain he had died. He burst out of his snow cave and said, "I am alive!"

This was a profoundly interesting story for me because it demonstrated how doing nothing really can save lives. Most people think doing nothing is just sort of a feeling, you know, it just floats around in your brain somewhere, above your clavicles, and doesn't do anything substantial. But it can be transformative.

Let me tell you another anecdote about the power of doing nothing, this one from Texas history. One of the explorers who followed Columbus to the new world was Cabeza de Vaca. He shipwrecked on Galveston Island and here he is, his ship is down, his crew mates have run away, he doesn't even have any clothes and it's December. To save his life from the Indians, he buries himself in the ground, stays there three days and nights, and when he emerges from the dirt he finds that a fantastic transformation has taken place. Cabeza de Vaca now has the power to heal. The thing that saved his life and allowed him to be able to walk westward without being harmed was that word of his healing power got out and proceeded him on his journey. The natives would bring their sick for him to heal. Here was yet another example of the transformative power of doing nothing, in this case an experience that allowed a man to discover his previously hidden healing abilities.

This state of emptiness, which is such an important part of this paradigm we're exploring, is viewed with enormous skepticism within our culture. We are taught always to be *doing*. I know people who are busy from the moment they put their feet on the floor in the morning to the time they turn the light off at night, filling their days with an endless procession of *doing*.

For so many people in the health movement, life is an unending search for the right formula, whether it's vitamins, herbs, diet, exercise, meditation, psychotherapy, personal development or what-not. We forget that we sometimes need to just kick back and not *do* but just *be*—and to wait patiently, as Jung once said, for whatever the universe wants to give us.

I remember this story now, that as Cabeza de Vaca came back to civilization, his healing powers disappeared because he felt he was getting closer to doctors who he believed knew more than he about healing.

Yes, when he turned south at El Paso, to go on to Mexico City, which was the seat of Spanish civilization then, two things happened. First, he lost not only his ability to heal but also his desire to heal. As he put it, everyone knew that Mexico City was where you found real doctors. This may be one of the first recorded incidences in western history of the split between medicine and healing.

Before we close, I'd like to ask you about the Planetree story because I think it's so important. Maybe you could just give us a quick rundown.

Planetree is a unit of about two-dozen beds at Cal-Pacific Presbyterian Hospital in San Francisco, where we perhaps catch a glimpse of the hospital of the future. At Planetree, everything has been done to change the meaning of the hospital experience.

It doesn't look like a hospital. All resuscitation equipment, bandage carts, etcetera, are out of sight.

What impressed me is that people who are able are encouraged to cook their own meals.

They can cook their own meals, even write in their own charts. They get to read their own charts. They get a library printout of all the current research on their own particular disease. Visiting hours are whenever the patient wants them. They can have their tests whenever they want them, and so on. This is a sensational effort. People feel empowered to take an active and constructive role in the healing process. It's a sign of the future.

The experience of being in such a situation could be very healing then, couldn't it, as opposed to the very disempowering process that we too often experience in more traditional hospital settings.

It is a move toward a new era in medicine, perhaps a small move but I think a significant one.

Section Two

Beyond Space and Time— Exploring the Non-Local Mind

Thanks to breakthroughs in physics, human consciousness research and medicine, there is now sufficient evidence that the mind is non-local, that is, it is not confined to the brain, not limited by the bony structure of our skulls or even by our physical bodies. In fact, it may very well be that our minds extend beyond the boundaries of all physical limitations, into a vast, infinite realm. Indeed, the techno-shamanic-physicists tell us everything within our universe is interconnected. As an old friend and mentor of mine, Joseph Campbell, once wrote: "The old Gods are dead or dying. And people everywhere are searching, asking, What is the new mythology to be? *The new mythology is of this unified earth as one harmonious being." Today, this is our quest, to explore the mind and the possibility of the existence of the soul.*

Larry, in your past books and lectures, you've made the case that medicine is a lot more than what we thought it to be. But you are now exploring the relationships between the spiritual and the medical. What led you to this. How did you get interested in this very challenging realm?

I began to look at data in my first two books showing that the mind really exerts a tremendous influence on the body's behavior where illness and health are concerned. I was caught up in this evidence as a great many other physicians were in the late 70's, early 80's. Gradually it became apparent to me that we are looking squarely at the emergence of a very new era in medicine. This evidence was staring us right in the face—that the power of the mind in healing is even more glorious than we were thinking. This goes beyond mind-body medicine, Michael. We gradually have accumulated evidence that there is some aspect of the psyche that not only can affect the body, as we thought, but which extends beyond the brain and the body, bursting the bonds of the here and now. This aspect of the psyche begins to look very much like our ancient concepts of the soul.

What we mean by the soul, at least in the west, is some aspect of ourselves that is infinite, beyond the limits of space and time. It is omnipresent and as such may well be immortal and eternal. We don't have an electronic device that we can hook up to people and objectively measure the existence of the soul but there certainly is empirical evidence which suggests that it exists. Based on this evidence, it appears that the soul not only exists but that it bursts the bonds of the brain and the body and is spread through space and time.

What relevance does this have in terms of health? In our previous interview, we discussed how there are many people who are highly developed in the spiritual realm, but who still get ill and even die of diseases like cancer, in spite of their inner work.

This is a very tricky point because there has been the implication that if you have enough psychotherapy, if you do your spiritual homework, then you shouldn't have to put up with physical problems. But it just doesn't appear to work like that. There is a different calculus of health that somehow seems to take over at a certain level of spiritual realization. And it's important to point this out because a lot of people who are adherents to the so-called "New Age" thinking believe that when we get on a spiritual path and begin to develop our wisdom and understanding, we should transcend all physical problems. As a result we begin to feel guilty when we develop cancer.

If we have cancer and we proceed with our lives in a spiritually responsible way, and the cancer keeps growing, we feel as if we have done something wrong. Maybe we haven't meditated hard enough, or we have not mastered some part of our spiritual practice. I think it's worth pointing out that it just doesn't always work out in such a rational, logical way; as much as we are learning, we don't yet know enough about the relationships between spiritual achievement and physical health.

Since you brought up the term New Age, maybe this is a good place to comment and reflect. This term is much misunderstood. What does it actually mean? What does it symbolize? What is your understanding of this term? Many people see it as channels and crystals and airy-fairy flakiness and so forth. But how do you see it?

I wish the term itself would just go away! I think it's very misleading. One of the ways that it is most misleading is that it anchors our thinking in a linear notion of progress; there is an old age, and now there is this new age. I think the idea of linear progress, strung out through time, is an erroneous, misleading way to conceptualize our lives. And the fact is that many of the so-called "New Age" concepts actually come out of a timeless continuum of spiritual insights and beliefs.

The practicality of this, when carried out into health and illness, is the misconception that physical health is something which can be acquired and lived into the future, *ad infinitum*. "New Age" as a term undermines the idea of timelessness. I would want to emphasize something we might call eternity medicine—the idea that health is not to be developed, as such, but is something that is inherent and implicit in the universe, in a kind of timeless non-linear way. Within this way of perceiving, the ideal would not be to *become* healthy, as we presently think of health development, but to simply set the stage for the manifestation of the underlying perfection, pattern and wisdom that's always inherent throughout the universe.

In Recovering the Soul, *you referred to different eras of medicine, giving them numbers, that is, era one, era two, and era three. Could you elaborate on those for us?*

Era one is what could be called *mechanical medicine*; this is the kind of medicine that physicians have practiced in the techno-scientific era. It includes surgery, the use of drugs, radiation, and so on.

Beginning about thirty years ago, however, era two medicine began, which many of us now call "mind-body medicine;" it is what we associate with holistic health, complementary medicine, or alternative medicine. Some people think that mind-body medicine is as far as medicine can go. What could be better than the mind affecting the body? But beyond that there is yet another era of medicine that we can see in the making right now; this era is not like these other two eras. It is what I call "non-local medicine." The reason that it's not local is that in this kind of medicine, this kind of healing, the mind, some aspect of the psyche, does things that brains and bodies can't do. Brains and bodies stay put in the present moment, in the here and now, limited by the physical form. In non-local medicine, you have mind working at great distances. You have mind shuttling back and forth between past and future. There is nothing in era one and era two medicine that is comparable to this.

Era three involves the long-distance effects of prayer, distant healing, shamanic healings, and long-distance diagnosis for instance. All of these observations call for a new era which can't be described in so-called local terms.

I'm reminded of the work of people like Kenneth Ring and Dr. Raymond Moody on the near-death experience. The implications of their work is that something larger than the brain and the body is involved in our lives. There have been so many near-death experiences reported, in which part of the person's consciousness leaves the body and the brain and stands outside time and space.

Yes. And let's look at an example that I think is particularly revealing. In 1944 Carl Jung had a heart attack and he had a series of what he called tremendous visions. These were your classic near-death experiences. In one of these visions he began to behave non-locally, that is, outside time, and he saw that his physician was about to die. As it turned out, the first day the physician allowed Jung to sit up on the side of the bed, as part of the recuperative stage, that very same day the doctor took to his own bed, shaking with chills and fever. He was dead in short order, from septicemia, that is, blood poisoning. So Jung's mind, in this near-death experience, had apparently ranged beyond the ordinary boundaries of time. And he foresaw with great accuracy what was going to happen. Studies have shown that these aren't rare events and you don't have to be a spiritual genius like Jung to have them.

Surveys have shown that sixty percent of people in this culture have had these kinds of experiences, with their minds behaving in non-local fashion, spanning the distance between past, present, and future.

Yet our society, as a whole, is not very supportive of these experiences, is it?

No, I'm afraid not, at least not at the present time. And actually, so many of the people who have these experiences tend, after their recovery from the illness or injury that may have triggered it, to lapse back into the old local ways of perceiving their existence. I would hope that one of the benefits of calling attention to this empirical data, supporting this behavior of the psyche, would be that people would begin to feel validated in these experiences. Unfortunately one of the requirements for thinking something is worthy of our respect in modern society is to have it verified by science. So if science can smile on this domain of experience, perhaps people would be more willing to acknowledge and value experiences of this sort.

In your book Recovering the Soul, *you in fact talk about this—the emergence of scientific verification for non-local experience. I am thinking particularly of your comments about the work of scientists like Schrödinger and Einstein and Bohm. Maybe you could talk about that.*

Yes, indeed. Schrödinger wrote a book back in the 20's in which he called attention to the concept of the *unbounded mind*, or what he called the *one mind*. He was so leery about publishing this material, because of the cultural attitudes of that time, that he held off for about thirty years before he allowed the book to come out. The statements in question were based upon his studies in quantum mechanics and Vedanta, India's ancient mode of wisdom. Schrödinger said that if what he had observed was true, then minds are essentially unbounded, and if unbounded there cannot be five billion minds walking around on the face of the earth today; there can only be one mind. He linked this with the vision of Vedanta. We realize today that his thinking is consistent not only with the ancient vision of the east but with the vision that has cropped up in western culture from time to time, particularly in modern physics.

Ironically, this idea of universal mind had a position of great respect in Medieval Europe. Some of the profound geniuses of the Christian tradition also held to it. So this is not just a product of eastern mysticism. For me, the fact that so many scientific geniuses of this century have held to this idea of non-local forms of consciousness has been a great inspiration.

I know that Gödel, a great scientist in his own right, also came to this concept of one mind, didn't he?

Yes he did. In fact, in a little known interview just before his death, Gödel opened up to the interviewer and said that this is the reality. He fully acknowledged his belief in the idea of the universal, one mind around the time of his death.

And Einstein?

Einstein expressed it in a different way. He certainly had the idea that his consciousness was connected with that of everyone else's, and because he felt this way, the idea of freedom of the will literally made no sense to him. Who is there to will? He had no idea of himself as a separate entity. He felt that he was hooked up with everyone else. You can imagine, he had great trouble grappling with this idea of freedom of the will. How, after all, if you are so intimately connected with the one mind can you possibly act out of pure free will?

David Bohm, who has been a guest on this program several times, also mentioned Einstein and his theory of the implicate and explicative order.

Yes, indeed. Bohm has clearly acknowledged the existence of one mind and he, as well as Freeman Dyson, who is also one of the preeminent physicists of our age, have acknowledged the existence of a penetrating mind that extends from the farthest reaches of the cosmos down to the levels of the subatomic particles. If you look around the world of science, you can see these gigantic intellects acknowledging this phenomenon not only on the basis of their personal experiences but through scientific observation.

We should say that this is the cutting edge of science. But perhaps it has not really penetrated mainstream science.

Well, we certainly can't dismiss these people as cranks! We owe most of our 20th century concepts in physics, or at least a good number of them, to these people—leading scientists such as Bohr and Heisenberg and Schrödinger and Einstein.

I think it's interesting to note that Einstein postulated the theory of relativity about 1905, and many physicists have built upon and extended his work even further. Yet, there are still researchers who continue to adhere to the old Newtonian-Cartesian model of the universe 75 years later. Someone once compared them to the flat-Earthers, who cling to beliefs that have long since been revised or disproven.

Yes. There certainly are some diehards out there. There are some people in prestigious positions in modern physics today who really hold out for the development of a Newtonian brand of physics all over again. There is this subliminal hope that we can get back to the mechanistic predictability that characterized Newton's vision of the way the world works.

Poor old Newton! He really got a bad rap, in a way, since he was himself a very spiritually minded person. He recognized there was much more out there than meets the eye.

I agree with you. We've been hard on Newton. We've taken only his vision of the universe as a giant machine and dismissed all his other thinking. After all, Newton felt that God penetrated the universe. Modern physics has really picked and chosen those ideas of Newton's that they have liked and have completely dispensed with his spirituality and his alchemical ideas.

The culture has not supported that part of his thinking, so he's been the victim of the modern world selectively presenting the facts, as it were.

I'm afraid you're right.

Larry, another example of non-local mind is your concept of prayer and healing. One of the interesting things about your explorations has been your finding actual scientific experiments that have been conducted around prayer.

Yes. And I must confess, Michael, that when I discovered these empirical studies, showing that prayer really works, I was blown out of the water. I thought that prayer could never be nailed down that empirically. But it can be, and has been.

I think one of the most stunning clinical experiments in modern medicine was done at San Francisco General Hospital by a cardiologist, Randolph Byrd. Byrd randomized 393 patients who came through the coronary care unit with heart attacks, or the presumptive diagnosis of a heart attack. Half of them got treated with traditional coronary care-type medicine; half got that treatment but were also prayed for. This was a double-blind experiment; doctors, nurses and patients didn't know who was or wasn't being prayed for. To make a long story short, when the data was analyzed, the prayed-for group was superior in many, many different ways. I can tell you that if the effect being studied was a new drug or a new surgical procedure it would have been heralded in our culture as a major medical breakthrough. People would have been lined up for blocks to get their hands on this stuff or to have this procedure performed on them. As it was, the study practically went unnoticed.

Overall, Randolph Byrd's study is an elegant piece of work. It is really a landmark, showing the effect of prayer.

Some of the other pieces of the prayer puzzle come out of a group called the Spindrift organization. For over a decade they have quietly and systematically done studies showing the ability of what they call "prayer practitioners" to influence the course of simple biological systems. They will pray, for instance, for one batch of germinating seeds and not for another, then measure the germination rate of these groups. They may pray for one yeast culture and not another, then measure the difference in the carbon dioxide produced. They come out with numerical data to measure their results, and nothing is subjectively evaluated.

These studies have shown beyond any doubt that prayer is effective. Moreover, the results are reproducible and I think they put prayer in a completely respectable category of therapy, as a potent mode of intervention. I've looked at this data and these studies and I'm very, very impressed.

If I might mention something related about prayer, one of the most interesting things that this Spindrift group has done is to study the difference between two prayer strategies. One they called "directed prayer," and the other "non-directed prayer." In directed prayer, for instance, if you are praying for a sick person, you give God the diagnosis as well as the treatment you want Him to do. You want the tumor to go away or the person to recover from the heart attack, for instance. But in the non-directed approach you simply pray "Thy will be done." You don't tell God to go in any particular direction. The data shows that both prayer strategies are effective but the non-directed approach is two to four times stronger than the directed approach. This will be of interest to a lot of listeners since people everywhere are being told that if your images and visualizations are going to be accurate or effective they've got to be highly specific. In other words, in cancer you've got to really tell your T and B cells what you want them to do, and you've got to make these very vigorous, robust clear images. This data suggests the opposite is true. It suggests that even though the highly directed approach works the most effective approach is this non-directed appeal to the universe, to God, to do what's right for the system.

I personally find this very appealing and I think many people will because there have been a lot of people I've talked to who feel a kind of relief to discover that it's not up to them to define the best outcome. It's not up to them to know what's best. Sometimes we can't know what's best. I've seen people almost celebrate when they discover non-directed approaches work better because they feel that this is best for them. It suits their spiritual aesthetic if you will. They're not taking the position that they know things that God doesn't.

Would you say there is an element of surrender in this kind of non-directed prayer?

That is an excellent way to describe what's happening. Other terms might be *alignment* or *attunement*. If you look at the kinds of prayer that have been recommended by people, in the writings of Meister Eckhart, for example, we find that they are all non-directed. And the Lord's prayer, "thy will be done," is itself a non-directed form. So I think there is good reason to rethink these recommendations about the specificity of prayer and imagery and visualization.

The implication of "thy will be done" is a key concept then. It is honoring the Higher Power, God, however one chooses to speak of It, above one's own will. To do otherwise is to presume that my needs and my perceptions are more accurate, more important than anyone else's—including God's. With the more directed prayer there's the underlying sentiment that God should save me no matter what.

Yes, and this non-directed strategy takes prayer out of the wish list category and puts it on a different plane that many people, I think, find a lot more comfortable.

So, do you think medicine will one day say to the cancer patient, here are the therapeutic choices: surgery, chemotherapy, radiation or prayer?

Well, I think we are going to offer both prayer and the other therapies. One term we might use to describe this new approach is *complementary therapy*, where we can use era one, era two and era three approaches. That is an important point—we joke about it, but I see patients in my practice who don't understand this; that they can use both or all three methods. When their prayer fails, for instance, they may have an attack of guilt, thinking that they've let down their higher self, let's say, or that the disease entity is more powerful than the soul.

In other words, they did something wrong or they have not gone far enough in their own development.

Sure. I'll tell you that, if before the day's end I have an attack of appendicitis, I may well ask you to pray for me, Michael, but I'm going to call the surgeon, too! So I want you both to do your jobs. I think this is not well understood among people who are interested in holistic approaches.

I don't want to lose this particular point—that the non-directed prayer approach allows a place for the notion that there is some inherent pattern and rightness and wholeness to the universe which I may not understand but which can manifest if we surrender, attune, align or simply get out of its way. These kinds of psychological and spiritual strategies seem to set the stage, in many instances, for the emergence of healing. And it's not something we actively do. It's more like an acceptance of a psychological emptiness or spiritual void if you will. If you look at the occurrence of miracles, and this has been done systematically, and you interview people who have experienced miracles, then it seems the people who are best set up for these miracles are those who are in a state of psychological attunement or alignment and are not specifying how God should do the work. There's a report by the Institute of Noetic Sciences on a trip they made to this pilgrimage site in Yugoslavia, where they interviewed people whose symptoms such as blindness or tumors have gone away as a result of their prayers at this site; you find some very interesting things. Father Slavko is the priest in this little village. Of all things, it turns out he has a Ph.D. in psychology and he has actually interviewed people who have undergone these spontaneous, radical unexpected healings. He says that these people are different. They are in an altered state of consciousness. They want healing or they wouldn't have come there in the first place. But healing, getting rid of the cancer or the blindness, is not their dominant motive. Rather, these people are standing on a stage of emptiness, attunement, alignment and surrender. The priest says that he can almost predict the people who are candidates for this kind of radical healing.

This is an important message to get across because a lot of holistic therapies these days are incessantly busy. They fill up every moment of waking space with techniques. People never turn off the willful doing. They never focus on the way of being. Even when meditation is done it's frequently done for a purpose, with a powerful goal in mind. When imagery and visualization work is done you always have that goal that you are trying to facilitate. A look at these radical healings suggests that there is another way to look at the process of healing through prayer, that it is not the *doing* that is important so much as the *being*, this surrender to the will of the universe rather than attempting to dictate to it.

I think this idea of imposing our will upon the universe, of constantly doing instead of being, permeates our culture.

Oh, precisely.

We've all been conditioned to believe that life is a linear track and we must go from one achievement, one goal to another. We forget the process of being that takes place between our achievements.

We are terrified of the spaces between achievements, of the periods of non-activity or non-productivity. We assume that these states are nothing more than a kind of hovering at the edge of the void. The void in this regard is nothingness, non-being, extermination, annihilation, death. We are extremely uncomfortable with that concept. Many other cultures, however, view the void as the plenum from which everything important comes. There is the idea that there's a pattern, an order behind the scenes that comes forward, makes itself better known to us when we stand before the void.

This idea has only in recent times begun to surface in many areas of science. In David Bohm's concept of the implicate order he describes something like a behind-the-scenes domain out of which everything manifests, arises. And there are areas in mathematics, such as in fractal geometry, where a hidden pattern is acknowledged. Chaos theory also suggests a pattern behind the scenes. Dissipative structure theory, whose theorist has already been awarded a Nobel Prize, also suggests that order can come out of sheer chaos and that chaos, in fact, has its own order. So even from modern science, let alone scrutiny of these miraculous healings, we see that what we call the void may frequently be the stage for the launching of incredible transformations—of chaos into order, of illness into health.

But where it gets tricky is that there is no apparent way to predict that these transformations are always going to happen. I mean this is not causality in the way we usually think about it. Bernadette, the young French peasant girl who saw the vision of the Virgin Mary and set the tradition at Lourdes in motion, did not herself have one of those miracles. So, you see, we are perhaps talking about something that is, as Jung called it, "acausal," that is, outside the causal realm. Just assuming this psychological state doesn't guarantee what we might judge to be a "good" outcome.

We must be careful about certain assumptions that we make in this regard—that we must not expect a contract, a guarantee of certain results when we follow the apparent guidelines that emerge from our observations here. The wise ones have never seen adherence to an apparent truth as a guarantee of freedom from illness and death on this physical plane. If you look at the way health and illness correlate with spirituality in the east and the west, there has never been a straight linear, cause-effect correlation implied or expected.

Earlier we were talking about a certain kind of New Age thinking, in which there is the implication that if you are sick there is something wrong with you psychologically as well as physically, that it is never just a physical thing. It must be that you don't have your act together because you have this physical problem. What about that?

I think the people who are saying this may very well be building up some very bad karma for themselves. I think that this way of thinking can do enormous harm. I like to line up with Jung on this point. He said that we cannot compel the unconscious into our little neat categories. We have to sit in the *mysterium*, as he called it, and put up with whatever form it manifests. And he was very, very, clear on this. Most people, when they discover a connection between mind and body, fall on that with utmost enthusiasm and try to compel the unconscious as well the conscious mind to perform, to jump through hoops, to make all of the diseases go away. It just doesn't work that way. And even, again, if we look at the lives of the spiritual geniuses it seems that when they achieve a level of high wisdom, the calculus, the criteria for what wellness is all about changes. They do not see their tumor or their painful death as evidence of an ethical or moral failure. But too often we don't get that concept. Anything less is deleterious and harmful, I think, a cruel message to be telling people.

One of the things you brought up in the book was the idea of shamanic contact as being another example of non-local mind.

If we take the shamanic lore literally, there are non-local manifestations of psyche written all over it. I think that it is quite unlikely that if shamanism was nothing more than a hoax it could never have lasted as long as it has. It's still alive and well, as anthropologists know. The shaman was good at finding the horse that was lost beyond the third range of mountains, telling people where the battle was going to be fought, where and when the rain was going to fall. These are all non-local manifestations of the psyche. Shamans know this world well. I really think that shamanic lore has really been a neglected source of evidence for the non-local manifestation of the mind.

What about communications with animals? In Recovering the Soul, *there is the story of a family moving from Ohio to*

Oregon. They had a pet collie dog named Bobby. Bobby had never been to Oregon though the rest of the family had. As they were going through Indiana Bobby ran off and got lost. They look for Bobby and can't find her. So they are compelled to go on to Oregon. Three months later there is a scratch at the door and there is Bobby at their new home in Oregon! How can we explain that? It can't be sheer coincidence. I mean it is just phenomenally too far-fetched. Shall we say that Bobby had telepathy and just knew at a distance how to get to the family's new home? Does your idea of one mind explain it? If we take the concept of one mind seriously, we have to say that if one element in that mind knows something, then it must also be available to everybody else who is a part of that mind, including animals. That's only one species. We could talk not only about dogs but dolphin research indicates that they can telepathically receive and send information, even across species. J. B. Rhine collected almost 60 cases of these strange returning animal stories, what he called psi trailing events. *They constitute, I think, an interesting part of the collective mind picture. It all heurkens back to Bohm's idea of the universe as holographic, that each piece of the universe is connected to the whole—and this certainly includes the mind.*

I think that's a powerful way to express it.

And in a hologram you can take any piece of the hologram and reproduce the whole.

Yes.

In your book you called St. Francis the patron saint of the non-local mind. Could you explain that?

Well, he took communication with animals seriously. He's been called by many of his biographers the severest heretic in Christianity since Jesus. He actually communicated with animals. He preached to the wolf, the wolf responded, and so on. He talked to the birds and so forth. And this was not just cute carryings-on. This was a felt connection, his biographers say. So I've said he would be a great patron saint for non-local mind because of these interactions, which depend on taking the one mind, the universal mind, completely seriously, which I think he did.

There is also the lore of the American Indian— that they would stalk their game and frequently, after encountering a herd of buffalo they would perform a particular ritual, making offerings to the buffalo, and then one buffalo would emerge from the herd, kind of electing itself as the ritual kill. There are other examples of stalking deer or a mountain lion, or whatever, actually merging or becoming one with the animal so that there was a shared mind, allowing the stalker to know his prey's every turn.

Yes, yes.

Isn't this another example of what you are talking about?

Exactly. It is probably true that the person who elevated the study of this collective mind to the highest level was Carl Jung. He resurrected this idea of the *anima mundi*, that is, the world soul. And he claimed, much as James Lovelock has, that there is a collective consciousness which envelopes everything on the Earth, that Mother Earth is not only alive, Lovelock maintains in his Gaia hypothesis, but that it is conscious. We can share thoughts with anything on this planet, and maybe beyond. So I find Jung's idea of *anima mundi* quite coherent with our concept of non-local, unbounded consciousness.

It's interesting because we have often criticized primitive societies for not developing higher technology or developing toward a more "modern" culture. But the fact is that if one looks at these cultures, generally, there was no need for them to develop higher technologies because they were already so in touch with their environment. I recall that scene in the film "The Right Stuff," based on Tom Wolfe's book by the same title. There was the story of this guy going to a tracking station in Australia and he was talking to some local Aboriginals who asked what he was doing, and he said, I'm tracking this space capsule up there in space. And they said, Oh, you're doing what he does, and they pointed to this Aboriginal shaman. He, also, traveled in space and knew the stars. It was true, the shaman knew as much as the astronomers did about the heavens. This was an example of the primitive and the modern coming together, with the primitive practicing non-local mind in your terms.

That's a beautiful example.

Larry, of course we have professional healers, people with M.D.'s after their names, and professional nursing practitioners and so forth. Then there is another category of healers that don't have the so-called credentials but nevertheless practice healing. Often, the latter are practitioners of non-local mind healing. Maybe you could talk a little bit about healers and healing.

Earlier, we mentioned the different eras in medicine, era one, two, and three, the mechanical, the mind-body, and then the non-local, such as is embodied in psychic or spiritual healing. I used to think that we ought to demand of our physicians that they be skillful in all of these areas. You know, you expect your doctor to be really adept at meeting your needs, whatever those needs may be. Recently, I've become sort of skeptical of that possibility, and I think that it's probably naive to demand that any single physician be able to bridge all of these different eras of healing, these different methodologies. For instance, in order to be a skillful era three healer, a psychic healer, a spiritual healer or shaman, this may involve a lifetime of spiritual effort, of spiritual growth. This is a path that extends over decades. I think that it is probably ridiculous to expect a young chap who is just out of medical school to have mastered this. It doesn't even work that way among the spiritual healers at that age. So, as much as we don't like the term these days, compartmentalization of the healing effort is probably necessary.

You know, we don't expect spiritual healers to do heart transplants; in the same way I doubt we can expect era one mechanical physicians to be effective with healing at a distance. What we can demand of them, however, is something we've never demanded and that is that they truly care and that they manifest love for their patients, even in the most mechanical medicine. I suspect that those are very potent factors. But as far as expecting single physicians to do everything, whether they are in the spiritual camp or the mechanical one, I think is probably unrealistic.

I think we also need to demand something we've never demanded of our spiritual healers—some sort of standard, if I might use the word. The Spindrift people have invited prayer practitioners to come and document their work with these simple experiments they do. And you know what the response was from the religious organization these spiritual practitioners were affiliated with? It was sheer hostility. They wouldn't participate. You know, when I became an internist I had to take board exams and be certified and demonstrate my skill. The Spindrift people were saying the same thing: Look, you're telling people you are a prayer healer, show that you can do what you claim you can do. So the practitioners really didn't like that and they came to blows over that issue. Personally, I think we owe it to our patients to somehow show that we can do these things. I think it's a matter of integrity and honesty regardless of whether you call yourself an era three, non-local based healer or an era one mechanical sort of physician. I think the same rules might apply in a similar way to all three eras.

I'm not saying these standards would be as easy to create for spiritual healers as they would for mechanical physicians. Almost certainly, they would not. But we should expect them to heal at least some of the time. I think that's not asking too much. Certainly there is not going to be the predictability and the causality in the spiritual domain as there is in the mechanical forms of healing. But we should at least expect some demonstration of competence.

Going back to an earlier part of our conversation for a moment, to our discussion of prayer and surrender and accepting our connection to a greater whole. Maybe an important part of this surrender and acceptance is that it may just be our turn to die and so that's what happens. The disease which we may perceive as a bad thing, something to fight, is just a part of a natural order of things, normal and healthy in the bigger picture. Given that this is so, healing might take on a very different character, that is, the healing might involve allowing the person to die, or assisting them in confronting the reality of death as a positive part of the whole. So healers may not always eradicate the disease in every single instance. And so, one has to accept this possibility as well, right?

Yes. I would have to agree with that.

In the medical establishment, there is a great resistance to alternative modes of healing. What about that? You've been through the medical system and are exploring the other side. You've literally lived on both sides of the fence. What are your observations about this resistance?

Well that's a touchy issue. There are some things going on people don't know very much about. You see the reason that physicians have wanted to maintain control over their patients and the reason they have manifested hostility toward alternative healers is a need for power. They want to keep everything to themselves. In many ways however, that approach has resulted in the wheels coming off modern medicine. Eighty-five percent of people perceive that it's wrong; they want a major change. And the interesting thing to me is that it has led to a situation of extreme pain for the healers themselves. Most people think physicians are pretty much in control. They make a lot of money, they have a lot of power. It is very little recognized that as a professional group, physicians are spiritually and psychologically in a lot of trouble these days. I cannot remember when on early morning rounds at a hospital I have heard a positive conversation between two doctors. Rates of drug addiction, alcoholism, divorce and so on are quite high, as everyone knows. The level of pain for the average M.D. in this culture is enormous!

You're saying this is the price doctors pay for their somewhat distorted position in our society.

Absolutely. Moreover, I think that it's going to be increasingly recognized that a source of that pain is this frenetic desire that doctors have to keep it all to themselves and to not let anyone else in on the show. Clearly, alternative therapists can take away a lot of the responsibility that physicians have always felt they needed. They can ease the burden and paradoxically doctors can be empowered by giving up power. It's difficult to get that across. But I think we are at a juncture in the healing tradition where that is going to be one of the major changes. And it's hard to explain that to physicians and I'm not able to do it even with my colleagues very clearly. But I see in their lives when they give up power it becomes easier for them and they become empowered in that process.

Clearly there has been some rapport, albeit not perfect by any means, but there is still a great deal of resistance to spirituality in the medical setting. You know, the priest can come visit, the minister can come visit. But one might envision the modern hospital of the 21st century, with era one, two, and three practitioners working together. There would be body-mind healers, prayer healers, working alongside medical doctors and along with the latest technology. They would share equally in the power and the responsibility of serving the larger whole, the one mind.

Actually, one of the leading futurists in medicine, Leland Kaiser, from the University of Colorado at Denver, has proposed already that we begin to treat patients at all these levels the moment they come into the hospital; those who have had experience with meditation and conscious relaxation would go to a ward where they would not only get traditional orthodox care but would have access to alternative healers who would teach them in those methods with which they already have some experience or expertise. Those people who have never done any of that would go to a different ward so they could learn about some of the choices available to them beyond strictly modern medicine.

Nearly two decades ago, there was a case published in the most famous medical journal in the world, the *New England Journal of Medicine,* in which an instructor of transcendental meditation was taken into the coronary care unit at Harvard's main teaching hospital, where he was successful in teaching this intractable patient how to meditate. I suspect if it's okay in Boston it can be carried into almost any other hospital. The effect of that combined coronary care unit and meditative approach was tremendously successful in that one instance.

In concluding this interview, might I ask you to reflect on the future of medicine and healing? How are we going to bring this new vision of yours into play?

Well, I think we are going to see continued growth of technology in medicine. I believe that goes without saying. But there is a difference. Part of the scientific thrust is going to be a new focus on these non-local methods of healing—the use of prayer, for instance. I predict that it will get to the point where if a physician does not invoke the alternative non-local approaches, it will be seen as malpractice as these forms of healing are increasingly proved to be potent interventions.

And we can all look forward to that day!

Section Three

Prayer, Science, and the Power of Healing

A Newsweek *cover story reported that 91 percent of all women pray, as do 85 percent of all men. Indeed more of us pray than have jobs or exercise or have sexual relations. There is an abundance of scientific studies supporting the effectiveness of prayer, published in journals mostly unread by physicians as well as patients. Even clergy and deeply religious people are uninformed about this information. We no longer need to take it on faith alone; the fact is that prayer works to heal. Larry, my first question to you is how do you define prayer? Is there a simple definition?*

I don't think there is. I was astonished in researching this whole area to go through dozens and dozens of books written by world class authorities on prayer where there was not a single definition offered for the subject of the book itself. This is quite an extraordinary situation.

I think that most people growing up in our culture probably think of prayer as talking to a white male cosmic parent figure who basically prefers being addressed in English. I'd like to paint the canvas a lot bigger, however, and define prayer in a different way. For me, prayer is any act that brings one in closer contact with the transcendent. It may involve words, but as often as not it involves silence, privacy. I don't think prayer necessarily even involves a waking, aware state. I am convinced that prayer can be deeply unconscious. There are some fabulous stories that have to do with healing events wherein people prayed in their dreams. So, prayer is a very complex way of communicating with something that is omnipresent. But all too many of us lock ourselves into a very narrow conception of prayer at the outset, in which we say that it necessarily has something to do with words. After researching this area for many years, I am convinced that prayer often does not involve words at all.

We don't usually associate prayer with the medical establishment, either. I mean, most hospitals don't emphasize prayer, unless they happen to be run by a religious order of some kind. But in your books and lectures you are talking about prayer as an integral part of medicine and the healing process. I have to ask, if prayer is so good, why has it almost been hidden away in hospitals?

Well, prayer is an embarrassment to most people in my profession, Michael. I don't know of any nicer way to put it. We can't acknowledge that it has any substance because of one primary reason; there is no "scientific" theory in modern medicine that even suggests that prayer is effective. Lacking a theory, most physicians feel compelled to say that since it isn't in the medical books, and isn't in the training, it isn't real, it doesn't work. This attitude, of course, really loads the dice against anybody looking at the empirical evidence. You're convinced ahead of time that any evidence supporting prayer must be flawed; that's the bias in medicine today. So if you're a physician and you value yourself as a scientifically inclined person, you'll think twice before you take the risk of standing up publicly in favor of prayer. It's easy to see why it is mostly ignored in medicine.

And yet, in your book, Healing Words *, you indicate that you found a lot of scientifically valid research that has revealed the power of prayer.*

There are studies that frankly knocked my socks off. Interestingly, I didn't get into this area voluntarily. I feel like I was basically dragged, kicking and screaming, into it, for one basic reason: I value science and I consider myself a sort of science junkie. These studies on prayer, which I stumbled onto, really shook me up. They lead to questions like: Look Dossey, you claim to be a scientifically-oriented person, what are you going to *do* with this information? Are you going to honor it? Are you going to let it into your life, into your work? Are you going to engage it? Are you going to let it make a difference in the way you practice medicine?

I think that the job of a medical scientist is to go *through* the data wherever it may take you and accept whatever violence it may do to your preconceived ideas about how the world ought to work. If you have to revise your own ideas then, well, you do that. I was reasonably shaken up by the discovery of this data. So, this information posed a profound personal challenge for me.

The thing that sets this book of mine apart from most books written on prayer is that few of them have acknowledged these controlled, prospective, clinical studies that have been conducted with the most stringent laboratory discipline. My challenge to my colleagues with this book is to say, "Look guys, here's the information. Let's play science together. Let's honor all this data because it is not going to go away. It's there to be dealt with. We no longer can ignore it."

Well, I'll bite. I'll play science with you. What are some of the more striking experiments you found?

Well, the first one that comes to mind is the study that we discussed in our previous interview, by Randolph Byrd at San Francisco General Hospital. You'll remember that he was working with cardiac patients, who'd recently suffered heart attacks or people who had severe chest pains, and he found there were fewer deaths in the group that was prayed for. There were other significant differences; for example, nobody in the prayed-for group had to be put on a ventilator to help them breathe, while twelve in the group not prayed-for required this. The statistical differences in recovery were so significant that if they had been evaluating a new medication or surgical procedure, it would have been celebrated as a medical breakthrough.

There are, in addition, a great many studies that do not involve humans. These have dealt with the effects of prayer on lower life forms such as bacteria, yeast, fungi, germinating seeds, mice, rats, ducks, baby gerbils—organisms that presumably are not susceptible to placebo phenomena. This is important since one of the criticisms that's always levied at these prayer experiments with humans is that somehow the subjects knew they were being prayed-for so that our positive outcomes are simply reflecting placebo responses. You can't accuse bacteria of having that sort of response. Presumably they don't know they've been prayed-for. Presumably bacteria and yeast and fungi are not subject to suggestion of the kind that would distort the scientific data in humans.

What do we find in these studies? Well, over half of them reveal that something stunning, something statistically significant, has gone on in the these creatures. Now, I'm talking about studies that have been performed at first-rate institutions, many universities, psychology departments, and independent research centers. They have been the subject of Ph.D. dissertations, masters theses and so on. There's a ton of data out there supporting the power of prayer in the healing process.

I wonder if one of the reasons we haven't heard more about these studies is that you can't put prayer in a pill and sell it. And it does bump up against the scientific view that it isn't real unless you can see it, touch it, feel it, smell it, or manipulate it. I suspect that if it could be validated in those terms, we might have a very different level of acceptance here.

Well, I think you're right. There are all sorts of financial disincentives involved when you are talking about it as a therapeutic factor. If you could package and sell it, it would be the ideal product, particularly because it has no contraindications and few side effects.

One thing that keeps it out of the scientific eye is a complaint that has been out there ever since Galileo accused Kepler of it—the belief in action at a distance. You know, if you want to say something really nasty about a scientific colleague, all you have to do is accuse him or her of believing in action at a distance. Prayer is action at a distance. There is no theory now accepted in modern science that says that anything could act at a distance with no energetic signal in between. But prayer apparently does work in a way that's unmediated. You can't block it. You can't shield it. It works as powerfully on the other side of the earth as it does an inch away.

And yet, in quantum physics we hear of wave and particle experiments in which wave turns to particle and vice versa through the influence of the observer. Here we have a phenomenon in which there's no visible or measurable connection—in short, science can't ignore the effects of what you're calling "action at a distance."

That's true. This area of science is alive and well these days, buzzing with insights and discoveries about "non-locality." So action at a distance is at home in the quantum mechanical world. Now whether or not this model will eventually explain how prayer works is open to question. Actually, a Nobel physicist, Brian Josephson, has proposed that quantum non-locality lies at the heart of non-local experiences people report at psychological, spiritual, and mental levels. There are some pretty heavy-duty researchers these days looking to quantum physics for explanations of how prayer and clairvoyance and telepathy might work. I must say this is all theoretical at this stage and whether it really proves to be the explanation for prayer remains to be seen.

You mentioned placebo affect—that prayer might produce a placebo affect. I'm thinking of all the scientific studies that have proven that placebos themselves can work, that they sometimes heal. They work, showing that belief itself can trigger the production of neurotransmitters in the body that, in turn, does the healing. So, let's say that prayer does trigger the so-called placebo effect; does that invalidate it as a healing method?

First, I'm sure prayer does generate placebo effects. If someone knows they are being prayed-for and they feel good about it, and they get some strong surge of neurotransmitters as a result, that perks up their immune system —and that's fabulous. Where this begins to really become even more interesting, however, is when the person is prayed-for at a distance and is completely unaware that he or she is being prayed-for, and then something good happens. How do you explain that? So that's where the rub comes, scientifically. I'm almost amused at the trouble that specialists and physicians have over explaining this problem. I think our job is to honor the findings of these experiments. If we have an explanation for how and why they work, that's terrific. If we don't, that's no excuse not to honor the results. Frequently in medicine the explanation comes later. This was so with penicillin. When penicillin was first discovered we didn't have a clue about how or why it worked. But it was obvious that it did. It took a long time to uncover the explanation. I think we are at the same state with prayer. We don't yet have an explanation that satisfies everyone. But that shouldn't justify our tossing out our observations. Our job is to go straight through the data and not skirt around it. We've got to engage it.

Larry, what about experiments in other cultures? Has there been any research in other countries on this subject?

Most other cultures aren't sitting around holding their breath and waiting to get the results of the latest double blind study. They just go about their praying. I know of no other cultures making such a concerted effort to prove the power of prayer through laboratory studies.

One interesting point has come up in this field and that is the question of whether or not the Almighty is involved in prayer. Most people in our culture tend to believe that a personal God, Goddess, or whatever you want to call Higher Power, is the real source of the power of prayer, that any benefits one might enjoy are the result of Her or Him hearing us and giving us what we want. There are other cultures, however, that do not believe in a personal god, yet prayer seems to work for them as well. The most notable example of this is Buddhism. Buddhism isn't a theistic religion. They don't hold to the notion of a personal God. But Buddhists pray like crazy. They go through life spinning their prayer wheels! And these prayers are answered, too. So it challenges us to ask, "Well, what do we do with the God concept? Is this belief in a personal god central to prayer?" Even with the Buddhists, of course, you can say, "Well, they believe in a God within. So that is the Absolute Power which answers their prayers." These points are fascinating from an anthropological point of view, and all of them come up in the process of designing research projects around the power of prayer. You also discover there are many people in our society who find it offensive to even discuss the idea of prayer without a personal God. Most don't like to hear that Buddhist prayers work just fine with no personal God included.

It reminds me of a Kabir line: "Many people know that the teardrop goes into the ocean; few people know that the ocean goes into the tear drop."

That's true.

Your point about God is interesting from another vantage point. It brings up this notion that something outside ourselves will take care of us. For Buddhists, as you point out, there is this belief that the power is within. Perhaps prayer catalyzes that power…

I completely agree with that. I recall Joseph Campbell saying that if you look at Christianity from a certain vantage point you can also come up with the idea of a God within. For instance, he pointed out that the Bible teaches that the Kingdom of God is within. Campbell went on to ask, "Who is in the kingdom? God is in the kingdom. So that means God is within." So maybe Christians and Buddhists are not so far apart after all. It has been difficult for modern Christians to buy into this idea of the Divine within. Throughout the history of Christianity, people who put forth this idea have been charged with heresy and blasphemy.

You had a chapter in your book Healing Words *about the dark side of prayer, that prayer can actually bring harm. What about that?*

Well if you want to think of prayer as a therapy—and a lot of people do use prayer as therapy—I've never seen a therapy under the sun that didn't have side effects. So we might automatically expect that prayer might have some side effects. On the basis of both people's anecdotal reports and the laboratory evidence, it seems that there is a dark side, a shadow side to prayer. It would appear, for example, that if the praying person in the laboratory experiment switches his or her emotions from a loving, empathetic, compassionate state, to one that is really negative or even hateful, the lab subject is affected negatively. Its growth is retarded, for example, and in some instances the lab subject has died. So you can demonstrate negative effects in the laboratory that correspond to negative psychological states.

If you look around the world, you can find some dramatic examples that people can use the mind to cause harm, even death, at a distance. The most smashing one I came up with was a custom in the Hawaiian tradition that is called the *death prayer* in which the Kahuna shamans would gather together on an island and actually pray for the death of a person on a distant island, who was completely unaware that this was going on. Now, in all fairness, we should say that they would never use these negative prayers unless the target of their efforts was raising some real stink in the society and would not listen to any other reason. They would basically dispose of him from a distance. The person would literally die. If I could enlarge on one of the more bizarre aspects of this particular phenomenon, the point should be made that this is not voodoo-hexing. Voodoo-hexing is a local thing. The victim is *informed* that the hex has been cast, and he or she cooperates in the process, both psychologically and physiologically. Voodoo-hex death is not an immune system event, it is a cardiovascular-type death. In the death prayer there is no cooperation since the victim doesn't even know the prayers are being made.

This is the same thing with the Jivaro, is it not?

Exactly. Actually Michael Harner, who lived with them for many years, confirmed that he saw this practice carried out there. Well, as it turns out, in Hawaii the victim of this death prayer always dies in the same way. This is a striking observation. It is by no means obvious that the victim ought to die in the same way but they do. The method of death is a dead ringer for a disease that currently exists in modern medicine for which we have no explanation. It is called the Guillain-Barré syndrome. The feet go to sleep, the toes become numb, the feet become paralyzed and the numbness and paralysis rise up from the lower extremities to the trunk. When it reaches the level of the diaphragm the victim can no longer breathe, suffocates and dies. Today, we regard this as a disease of unknown origin, unknown etiology. We put people on mechanical respirators and keep them alive until this disease goes away. But we have no explanation for what causes it. It may be—and if somebody locks me up in an insane asylum for anything in this book, it may be this—that this particular disease, and maybe others of unknown origin, could be due to negative, psychological, non-local effects. In general, we might call these phenomena "psychic pollution." They have been recognized in perhaps every culture that has ever existed, except our own, where we are convinced that every disease has a physical explanation.

You know I'm thinking of places I've been in my life when I had the feeling there was something evil around and I just wanted to get out of there as fast as I could. There's the sense of it being in the air, in the emotional or spiritual space we occupy.

That's right.

I think of Sheldrake's morphogenic field theory and the concept of morphic resonance, the idea that the energy around a particular physical body, or the energy associated with a particular event, stays in the area, lingers for a time, sometimes for quite a long time. So maybe if something evil did happen in this place, what we are sensing is the morphogenic field of that event, still lurking around?

I take this possibility quite seriously. I live in a part of the world where there is a shaman on every corner: northern New Mexico. I have stopped asking them if they believe in these negative influences. They all say yes. I've begun asking them what they do to protect themselves. They have tremendously interesting protective mechanisms, as all pre-modern people do, to guard against this stuff. For us in the modern world, who don't believe in such phenomena, it wouldn't occur to us to take protective action, and so we are quite susceptible to these negative distant influences.

So how do we protect ourselves from these negative influences?

I could give you a couple of examples.

Please.

I have a friend in Santa Fe who is a very powerful shaman. Her name is Sandra Ingerman and she studied shamanism with Michael Harner. Sandra wrote the book *Soul Retrieval*. Her way of guarding against these influences is to say, "I refuse to participate at this level of reality. I won't engage with anybody who wants to try to duke it out with me spiritually." In other words, Sandra refuses to play the game. This apparently works beautifully for her. I have another friend in New Mexico, who is also a powerful shaman, and she goes about this entirely differently. She uses symbolic and concrete ritual. She has mirrors suspended from the four corners of her house; they twist in the wind and reflect things that could come her way. She also uses certain images. She imagines, for example, that she is coated one-inch-thick with lubricating jelly, and she says anything will slide off that. So you see, here you have this spectrum of protective mechanisms that people use; practically every culture, except our modern, scientific one, has ways of protecting themselves against these invisible attacks.

Yes. I think of Bali, for example, where they have these black and white checked umbrellas covering the local protector statues which you find in front of houses. The black and white checks are believed to ward off evil spirits.

And this would be viewed only as empty superstition in our society.

In recent years, Larry, our society has opened up more and more to the concept of the human soul. A decade ago, there wasn't a popular book on any publisher's list that talked about soul. Today, we have seen a number of books on this subject get on the New York Times *bestseller lists. Is this perhaps the indication of a change in our society, that people basically realize that we have neglected this area of life and are seeking to bring it back into their lives?*

Oh, absolutely. I think the major pay-off from our research into the power of prayer may go beyond the resolution of illness. If the cancer goes away or the heart attack gets better, that's great, that's a blessing, it's a grace. But I think the major benefit of the fact that prayer works has something to do with the soul. The fact that there is some aspect of the human psyche that can reach out at a distance—that can transcend spatial separation, that can go beyond temporal limitation—suggests that there is something about us that is soul-like, that has soul quality. The soul as we define it in the west is a quality of who we are that is infinite, existing outside the perceptual realities of space and time. You can't confine it to points in space, such as in a particular place in the laboratory or even in an individual brain or body. You can't even say it exists within the confines of a particular moment. In *Recovering the Soul* I attempted to describe that most essential aspect of who we are as "non-local."

I think we are now in a position with this research to say that we have reasonable, empirical evidence for the existence of the soul. For my money, this is such a sensational recognition that we ought to be shouting this from the rooftops. I think this is a big breakthrough, also, for addressing the fear of death. The evidence suggests that there is something about us that has no intention of dying when the body and brain die and rot. Part of us is immortal and unlimited by space and time. If the disease goes away, fine. But it hardly matters in the larger context.

Unfortunately, most people are blind to this majestic implication of prayer, they want to use prayer only in a totally utilitarian context.

How do you mean?

Manly P. Hall once said that there is a type of person who is always getting God mixed up with vitamins. They take a vitamin just to get healthier and would use prayer in the same way. I think that's fine in many respects. But there is an issue beyond whether or not the disease gets healed. Don't get me wrong; I'm all for that. All my professional life I have stood up for that position. But again, there's more to it than simply annihilating the disease. Sometimes we need to go through the disease and not be distracted by what the Buddhists have always called *attachments*. It's easy to get attached to the goal of perfect health, for example. It's easy to get attached to prosperity, to having a perfect relationship, or whatever else we might seek. Let me express this in a Buddhist teaching story:

In this parable, the student has been meditating the entire week and he comes to the Master and says: "Master, this is wonderful. I'm seeing white light. I feel at one with everything."

And the Master replies: "That's okay, just keep meditating. It'll go away."

The lesson here is that it's wonderful to experience these things—but beyond the pyrotechnics, beyond the sensations, there is something more fundamental, something that goes beyond the dichotomy of health and illness, beyond the dichotomy of prosperity and poverty, beyond bad relations and good relations. The central point is that we have something of the Divine within us that is already perfect the way it is. Our goal as human beings is to do the spiritual work that's required to wake up to this recognition.

It's interesting that the root meaning of the word "utopia," is a Greek root meaning "not in a place." That is, utopia is a non-local phenomenon, outside space and time.

Since it is not limited by time or space, it is right here, right now, in the present, always. *We're it!* At some level that's the goal of spiritual work. It's to realize that our "getting better" is not the point. The real point is to recognize that we are perfect already.

There was a time in my life when I was studying what prayer was really about and I read a description of how to pray. It said that while you were praying you should imagine yourself already fulfilled in whatever you were asking for. The idea was to hold in your mind the quality of the experience you would have when your prayers are answered, and then let go. Detach yourself from it. As I think about this now, I am also reminded of a Ziggy cartoon, where Ziggy is praying in the middle of the cathedral and he is saying, "Why me?" The roof of the cathedral opens up and a huge, bearded face peers down from the sky and bellows at him, "Because you bug me!"

You know, it's such a graphic, if amusing look at how most of us view prayer—that there is this superior person, or being, somewhere outside us, which we are either pleasing or displeasing, and who will bestow his or her gifts upon us only if we behave in a particular way and please this Higher Power. It's all a very external process, and there's a right and wrong way to do it—to pray.

That's right. That's exactly right. There is no particular formula for praying, and I think the point can be made that prayer is not directed to a particular being or power in the universe that we can presume to define, or have a mental picture of. It is helpful, I think, to look at the idea of utopia, that it is all here right now, in the here and now, and our souls are not limited by space or time, not limited by this particular body or mind.

There is a famous woman who wrote a book on prayer, Dr. Ann Ulanov. She once gave a lecture on prayer and a woman in the audience asked: "Dr. Ulanov, how should I pray?" Dr. Ulanov answered: "It is so simple, ask God." The lesson is, don't look at the books, don't look for special formulas, don't look to science, don't look to the laboratory. Look to God, Goddess. Turn inward, upward, inside out, upside down, where ever it is you go for those kinds of answers. That's where you will find how to pray.

One of the particularly intriguing chapters in your book Healing Words *had to do with the attitude of the healing professional, that this can actually have an effect, positive or negative, on the results of any medical procedure or any healing. That point really makes me realize that I should be much more conscious of who I choose to work with as a healer or medical professional. I would think it would have some impact on healers themselves as to the responsibility they carry in the partnership of the healing process with the client.*

There are research studies that show that if a doctor has doubts about a particular therapy that is being studied, these doubts or negative beliefs may actually penetrate the double-blind design and influence the outcome of the experiment. Here we are talking about action at a distance, non-local events if you will, where the thoughts and feelings held in the physician's mind can actually influence the outcome of a perfectly designed double-blind study. Researchers don't want to think about this, of course, because it suggests the awful possibility that the double-blind study is no longer the infallible standard we've always thought it to be. If doctors' pre-existing ideas can influence the outcome of double-blind studies, where are we? We may have to go back and reassess a lot of medical data. But to return to your original point, yes, we must be very careful about who we choose to enter into a healing relationship with, because a doctor's thoughts may actually influence the effectiveness of the therapy he or she prescribes.

Often, in my own experience, doctors seem to take the position of, "Oh, whatever works is fine." There is no commitment, as if they see the power only in the procedure or the drug that happens to be involved, and that's all there is to it. I mean, like that's not much of a commitment to healing. My experience is that a great many doctors take that position. How do you think it's going to change?

It will change the way the physicist Max Planck said physics changed. He said, around the turn of the century, that science changes funeral by funeral.

You're saying that sometimes you have to wait for your enemies to die off.

Yes, there is a lot of truth in this. But we want it to change quicker than that, and I am hopeful that it will do so. If you talk to a lot of the younger doctors, particularly women who have gone into medicine recently, they basically don't see things the same way; they are not the *old guard.* Their world view is changing medicine before our eyes. In addition, the fact that the whole health care system is in a state of crisis, a state of flux, is a hopeful sign. Sometimes the wheels have to come off before you can change the design of the wagon. But the main thing that makes me hopeful is the scientific evidence. You can't wish it away. This genie is never going to be stuffed back into the bottle. For instance, the new studies on prayer are critically important. They point to new forms of healing and to new concepts of the nature of the mind.

The most powerful metaphor in this culture is science. If we want to change our system of healing, the quickest way to do it is to come up with some compelling scientific evidence for alternatives. Whether we like it or not—and I must say I'm not particularly happy about this—science is a dominant force in our culture. If we go through it and honor the methodology I think we can effect radical and extraordinary change.

In point of fact, the research cited in your book is doing that, isn't it?

Yes, that's the whole point for bringing it up.

So what we are hopeful of seeing is more books—more doctors—coming forth to say, "Let's use prayer."

We're not going to see doctors waking up overnight *en masse*. What we *are* going to see is medicine changing because of pressures and developments, not so much from the inside, but from the outside. For example, most of the people who have produced the evidence supporting prayer are not on faculties at major medical schools. Mostly, they are working at the fringes of science. If you look at the pressures that were exerted to form the Office of Alternative Medicine at NIH a while back, you see that they were from people demanding alternative methods of therapy. This office was not established because people became enlightened within the National Institutes of Health. The potent pressures are coming from renegade scientists on the margins of science, and from regular folks.

So, how do you see this prayer thing going? I mean obviously it seems on a very positive track now with the work you have done and other research work you report in your books. But how do you see its future unfolding? Will it ever be integrated into mainstream medicine?

Let me re-state a prediction I made in *Healing Words.* There is already so much data supporting the positive effects of prayer in the laboratory and this data is only going to increase. As a result, prayer will become established as a legitimate practice in the community and ultimately, the doctor who fails to at least recommend prayer to his patient could be proven guilty of medical malpractice and sued. I think we are going to see a revolution around Prayer Therapy in this culture in the very near future.

That is an extraordinary prediction.

Biographical Notes on Michael Toms

Michael Toms is recognized as one of the leading spokespersons of "new paradigm" thinking. He has been a writer, book editor, scholar and broadcast journalist for more than two decades and is the recipient of two honorary doctorates for his ground breaking work in media. His perspective has been influenced greatly by his work with the late Joseph Campbell and Buckminster Fuller. He is perhaps best known as the host and executive producer of the widely acclaimed and award-winning "New Dimensions" national public radio interview series. He is Chairman Emeritus of the California Institute of Integral Studies, and currently serves as Senior Acquisitions Editor with HarperCollins San Francisco. His previous books include the bestselling *An Open Life: Joseph Campbell in Conversation with Michael Toms* and *At the Leading Edge: New Visions of Science, Spirituality and Society.* His interviews with leading thinkers of our time are the subject of our extensive "New Dimensions Books" series, edited by Hal Zina Bennett.

About New Dimensions

Inspired by the need for an overview of the dramatic cultural shifts and changing human values occurring on a planetary scale, New Dimensions Foundation was conceived and founded in March 1973, as a public, nonprofit educational organization. Shortly thereafter, New Dimensions Radio began producing programming for broadcast in northern California. Since then, more than 4,000 broadcast hours of programming intended to empower and enlighten have been produced. In 1980, "New Dimensions" went national via satellite as a weekly one-hour, in-depth interview series. More than 300 stations have aired the series since its inception, and "New Dimensions" has reached literally millions of listeners with its upbeat, practical, and provocative views of life and the human spirit.

Widely acclaimed as a unique and professional production, New Dimensions radio programming has featured hundreds of leading thinkers, creative artists, scientists and cultural and social innovators of our time in far-ranging dialogues covering the major issues of this era. The interviews from which this book was compiled are representative.

As interviewer and host, Michael Toms brings a broad background of knowledge and expertise to the "New Dimensions" microphone. His sensitive and engaging interviewing style as well as his own intellect and breadth of interest have been acclaimed by listeners and guests alike.

New Dimensions Radio provides a new model for exploring ideas in a spirit of open dialogue. Programs are produced to include the listener as an active participant as well as respecting the listener's intelligence and capacity for thoughtful choice. The programs are alive with dynamic spontaneity. "New Dimensions" programming celebrates life and the human spirit, while challenging the mind to open to fresh possibilities. We invite your participation with us in the ultimate human adventure—the quest for wisdom and the inexpressible.

For a free *New Dimensions Journal,* including a list of radio stations currently broadcasting the "New Dimensions" radio series, or an audio tape catalog, please write New Dimensions Radio, Dept. AB, P.O. Box 410510, San Francisco, CA 94141-0510; or you may telephone (415) 563-8899.

New Dimensions Tapes with Larry Dossey

Consciousness and Medicine with Larry Dossey, M.D.

In his startling book *Space, Time and Medicine,* this Dallas internist draws upon the discoveries of modern physics, which almost daily turns up new ways of understanding the universe, and relates these new understandings to health and healing. In this conversation Dossey shows us how new concepts of time and space—and a newfound role of individual consciousness—are revolutionizing health care.

Tape #1710 1 hr. $9.95

Visions of Wellness with Larry Dossey, M.D.

Thought-provoking and practical, Dossey questions the current model of health with its "body parts" orientation and presents new possibilities for medical care and disease prevention. using the contemporary insights of quantum physics as well as the ancient wisdom of time honored philosophies, he probes the meaning of health and the personal responsibility each of us has for our own welfare. The experience of health underscores this dialogue as Dossey adds new meaning to the search for wholeness.

Tape #1954 1 hr. $9.95

Physics, Medicine and Religion with Larry Dossey, M.D.

The evidence suggests that we are at some level unbounded in space and time, that we are omnipresent, infinite and immortal; and in this dialogue Dossey, a physician and writer, points to the nonlocal nature of the human mind. He explores the relevance of nonlocal mind to health and mentions some especially provocative research on the positive aspects of prayer as related to healing. For anyone wanting to understand the future direction of medicine or to probe the deeper possibilities for self-healing, this conversation provides a wealth of insight.

Tape #2193 1 hr. $9.95

Meaning Therapy: Medicine of the Future with Larry Dossey, M.D.

"We should look at meaning as seriously as we look at the cholesterol level or the blood pressure," says Larry Dossey as he explains a revolutionary concept in medicine. "Meaning therapy is a very powerful form of intervention, and we'll be seeing more of it in the years ahead." He envisions the medicine of the future as including compassion and emotional involvement on the part of physicians, and involvement and meaning-full awareness on the part of the patient. Through stories and compelling arguments he shows the importance to health of such factors as job satisfaction and symbolic meaning, but warns against overly simplistic interpretations of the profound and complex power of the unconscious. "Meaning enters the body," he says, "and makes the difference, in many cases, in life and death."

Tape #2299 1 hr. $9.95

Medicine, Meaning and Prayer with Larry Dossey, M.D.

These are exciting times in science and medicine, and Larry Dossey is a physician at the forefront of new developments on the interface of body and "soul." prayer, it seems, is holding its own in laboratory research despite the scientific assumptions it challenges. Dossey presents and evaluates the evidence, and explores its implications for both medical practice and individual healing. he goes even further, to an awareness of the deeper meaning of prayer and soul. Warning against "confusing God with vitamins" (seeing prayer as a tool for narrow practical ends), he reminds us of the larger context implied by the existence of soul, and the effectiveness not only of prayer but of non-attachment to results. A revealing and stimulating discussion for anyone with or without religious beliefs or skepticism.

Tape #2422 1 hr. $9.95

You are a vital part of the work we do!

Please become a member of "Friends of New Dimensions."

We encourage you to become a member of "Friends of New Dimensions" and help bring life-enhancing topics and ideas to the airwaves regularly. As an active member at the individual level or higher, you will receive:

- *New Dimensions* newsletter/journal, a quarterly publication containing feature articles and interviews spotlighting some of the same people and ideas you hear on our radio program, up-to-date program listings for the entire country, descriptions of new tapes, music and book reviews, and items of special interest to New Dimensions listeners.
- A 15% discount on all purchases made through New Dimensions.

Your membership contribution makes it possible to bring life-enhancing topics and ideas to the airwaves regularly, so please join at the level most consistent with your life- or work-style.

Use the order form on the following page. ➪

New Dimensions Order Form

(U.P.S. cannot deliver to P.O. box) Date ______________

Name ______________________________

Address ______________________________

City ______________________ State ________ Zip ________

Phone ______________________________

Tape #	Qty.	Title	Amount
1710		Consciousness and Medicine	
1954		Visons of Wellness	
2193		Physics, Medicine and Religion	
2299		Meaning Therapy: Medicine of the Future	
2422		Medicine, Meaning and Prayer	
	1	Tape Catalog	**FREE**

Subtotal	
15% membership discount	
Sales Tax — Calif. res. 7.25% BART counties 7.75%	
Shipping & Handling	
Membership	
Total	

Check type of payment:

☐ Check or money order ☐ Visa ☐ MC
(payable in U.S. funds)

____
Acct. #

____
Exp. Date

____
Signature—required for all credit card purchases

☐ **YES!** I want to support the radio work and become a member of "Friends of New Dimensions." I understand this entitles me to a 15% discount on all purchases from New Dimensions.

☐ Individual $35 (S721) ☐ Radio Council: $250 (SP 72)
☐ Family: $45 (S721) ☐ Satellite Sponsor: $500 (SP59)
☐ Sustaining: $50 (SP94) ☐ Benefactor: $1000 (SP95)
☐ Radio Underwriter: $100 (S726)

Send order to:
New Dimensions Tapes
P.O. Box 410510
San Francisco, CA 94141-0510
Or order by telephone:
(415) 563-8899
with VISA or MasterCard
ANY TIME, DAY OR NIGHT

SHIPPING & HANDLING

If subtotal falls between	add: U.S. & Canada	Foreign
0-$15.99	$2	$6
$16-$30.99	$4	$8
$31-$50.99	$5	$10
$51-$70.99	$6	$12
$71-$100	$7	$18
over $100	$8	$25

All domestic orders are shipped 1st Class mail or UPS. All orders going outside the U.S. are shipped air. FOREIGN ORDERS: Please send an international bank money order payable in U.S. funds, drawn through a U.S. bank.

OUR GUARANTEE: All New Dimensions tapes are unconditionally guaranteed. If for any reason you are dissatisfied, you may return the tape(s) within 30 days of purchase for a full refund or exchange.

Allow one to three weeks for delivery. AB

Other Titles in the New Dimensions Books Series

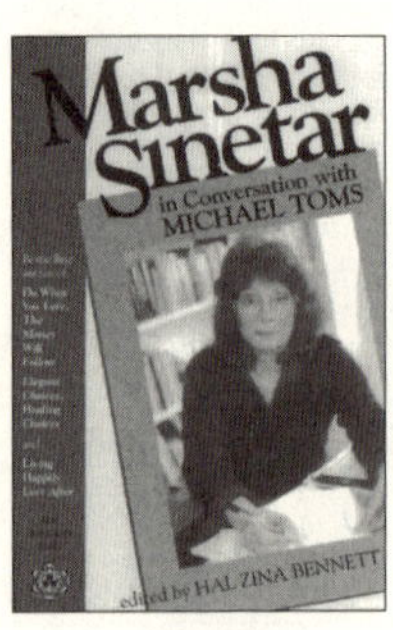

$8.95

Marsha Sinetar
in Conversation with Michael Toms

edited by Hal Zina Bennett

Marsha Sinetar is the best-selling author of *Do What You Love, The Money Will Follow* and *Living Happily Ever After.* In her work as an organizational psychologist, she has studied many people who have become successful doing what they love. In this new book, she speaks to those who are attempting to live their deepest calling in the midst of a seductive society. She emphasizes that choosing a lifestyle which blends inner truth with work, family and the demands of twentieth century life is more than possible—it's essential!

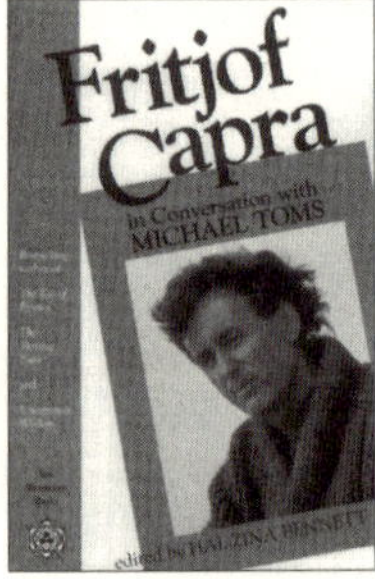

$8.95

Fritjof Capra
in Conversation with Michael Toms

edited by Hal Zina Bennett

In this book, Fritjof Capra takes us with him on his remarkable personal journey into the nether realms of quantum physics, where the traditional worlds of science and spirit twist and merge to the point where the distinctions become blurred. As he relates his wisdom-packed interactions with some of the leading contemporary thinkers and visionaries, from Gregory Bateson to Krishnamurti, we discover with him new ways of thinking and being.

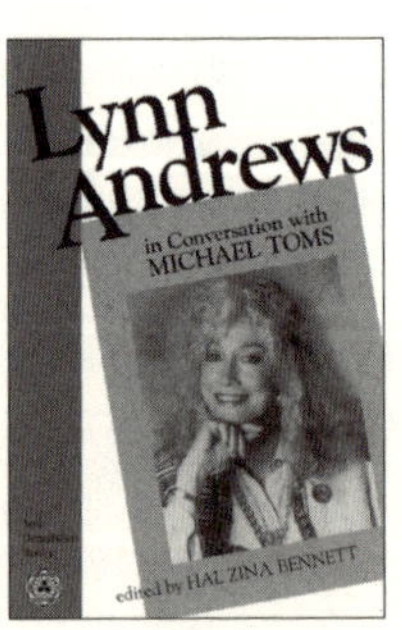

$8.95

Lynn Andrews
in Conversation with Michael Toms

edited by Hal Zina Bennett

Shamaness Lynn Andrews takes us into the wilderness of self to plumb the depths of our heart so that our being can soar. Her vision quest journey has taken her from the wilds of Manitoba to the jungles of the Yucatan and the Aboriginal outback of Australia, as she attempts to bridge the gulf between the primal mind and contemporary life. In this book, she challenges us to see the infinite range of possibilities that lies beyond our ordinary limits, and the planet.

Upcoming Books in the Series:

Patricia Sun in Conversation with Michael Toms

Anne Wilson Schaef in Conversation with Michael Toms

Other Books from Aslan Publishing

Gentle Roads to Survival

by Andre Auw, Ph.D.

This is one of those rare, life-changing books that touches the reader deeply. Drawing from his forty years of counseling as a priest and a psychotherapist, Auw points out the characteristics that distinguish people who are "born survivors" from those who give up, and teaches us how to learn these vital skills. Using case histories and simple, colorful language, Auw gently guides us past our limitations to the place of safety and courage within.

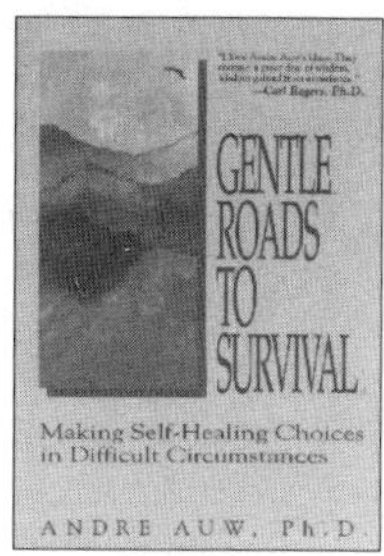

$10.95

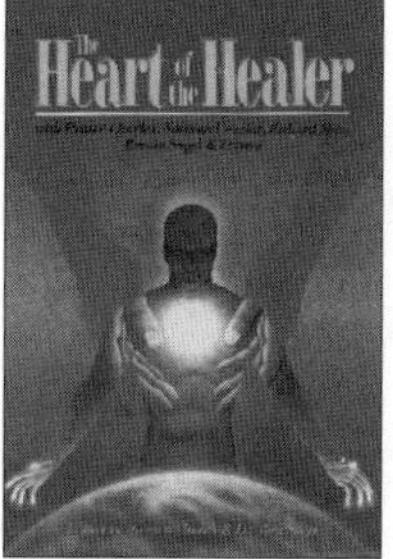

$14.95

The Heart of the Healer

edited by Dawson Church and Dr. Alan Sherr

Bernie Siegel, Larry Dossey, Norman Cousins and sixteen other healing professionals here intimately describe their vision of the healing process and the innermost workings of the true healer. An inspiring and definitive review of the emerging holistic paradigm in healing.

Intuition Workout

by Nancy Rosanoff

This is a new and revised edition of the classic text on intuition. Lively and extremely practical, it is a training manual for developing your intuition into a reliable tool that can be called upon at any time—in crisis situations, for everyday problems, and in tricky business, financial, and romantic situations. The author has been taking the mystery out of intuition in her trainings for executives, housewives, artists and others for over ten years.

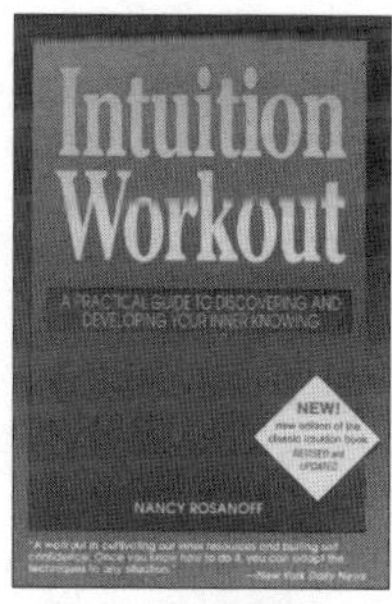

$10.95

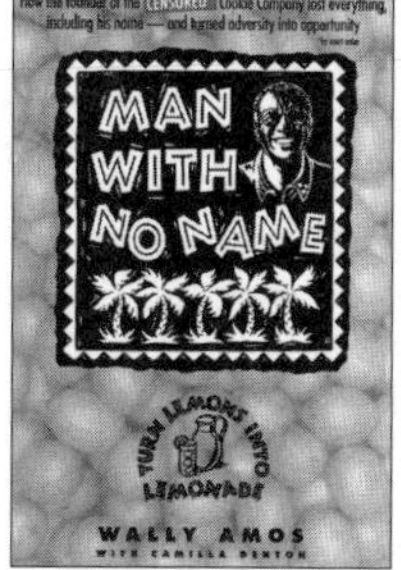

$9.95

Man with No Name

by Wally Amos

In his new book *Man with No Name* Wally Amos tells of his ordeal in losing his company, his slide into financial difficulty, the tribulations of a nineteen-month lawsuit, and the principles that kept him optimistic and ultimately victorious in the midst of seemingly desperate circumstances. Amos offers an inspiring and refreshing mixture of street smarts and spiritual faith, celebrating the triumph of the human spirit over adversity.

Other Books from Aslan Publishing

Living At the Heart of Creation

by Michael Exeter

Author Michael Exeter is one of the most important voices today for the emerging field of eco-spirituality. *Living At the Heart of Creation* pierces beyond the superficial fixes to the most pressing problems of our day. Blending profound spirituality with wide ecological knowledge, it offers remarkable insights into such challenging areas as the environmental crisis, business, relationships, and personal well-being, inspiring us to live at the heart of creation.

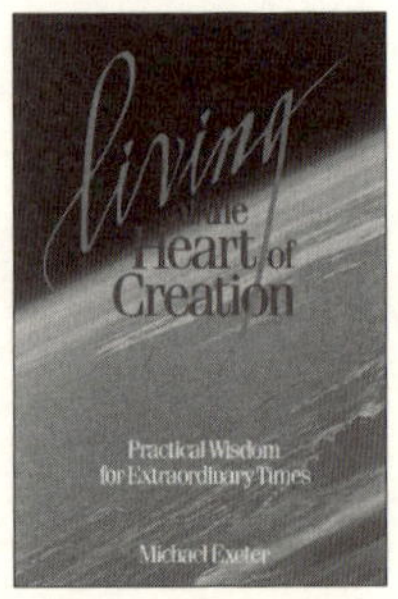

$9.95

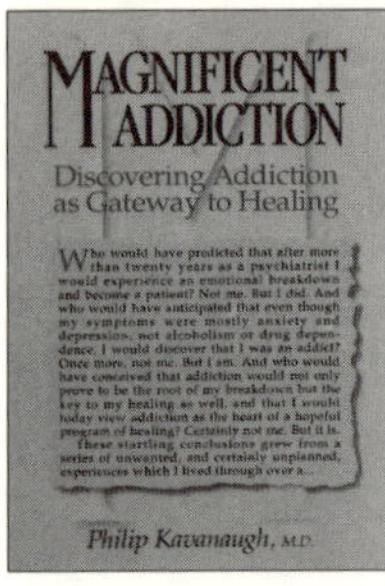

$12.95

Magnificent Addiction

by Philip R. Kavanaugh, M.D.

Kavanaugh's revolutionary work is decisively changing the way we see addictions and emotional disorders. Our unhealthy addictions aren't bad, he says—and it's a waste of time and effort to get wrapped up in getting rid of them, as he demonstrates in his own wrenching personal story. We simply need to upgrade our addictions to ones that serve us better, like addiction to wholeness, life, spontaneity, divinity.

Personal Power Cards

by Barbara Gress

An amazing tool for retraining the negative emotions that sabotage most attempts at recovery and personal growth, *Personal Power Cards* work scientifically through colors, shapes and words to re-program the brain for maximum emotional health. Called "One of the most useful recovery tools I have seen" by *New Age Retailer*, these are a simple, incredibly quick and effective technology for building a powerful sense of self-worth in a wide variety of life areas.

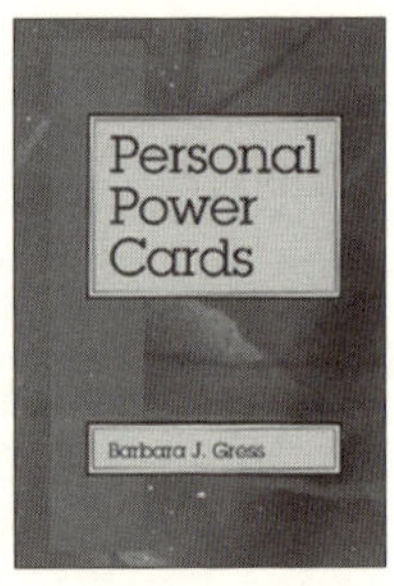

$18.95

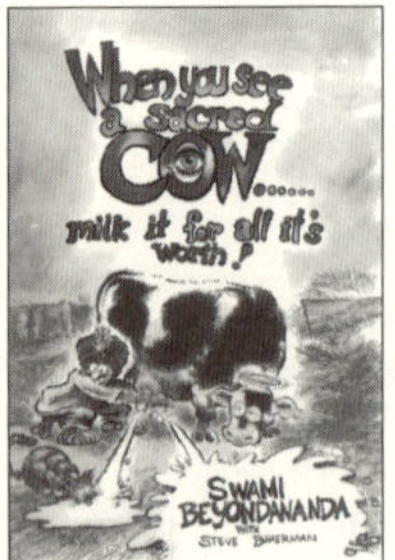

$9.95

When You See a Sacred Cow... Milk It for All It's Worth!

by Swami Beyondananda

The "Yogi from Muskogee" is at it again. In this delightful, off-the-wall little book, Swami Beyondananda holds forth on the ozone layer, Porky Pig, Safe Sects, and the theology of Chocolate. Read a few lines and you'll quickly realize that nothing's safe from his pointblank scrutiny.

Aslan Publishing Order Form

(Please print legibly) Date ____________

Name ______________________________

Address ______________________________

City ____________________ State________ Zip ______

Phone ______________________________

Please send a catalog to my friend:

Name ______________________________

Address ______________________________

City ____________________ State________ Zip ______

Item	Qty.	Price	Amount
Marsha Sinetar in Conversation with Michael Toms		$8.95	
Fritjof Capra in Conversation with Michael Toms		$8.95	
Lynn Andrews in Conversation with Michael Toms		$8.95	
Gentle Roads to Survival		$10.95	
The Heart of the Healer		$14.95	
Intuition Workout		$10.95	
Man with No Name		$9.95	
Living At the Heart of Creation		$9.95	
Magnificent Addiction		$12.95	
Personal Power Cards		$18.95	
When You See a Sacred Cow, Milk It…		$9.95	
		Subtotal	
		Calif. res. add 7.5% Tax	
		Shipping	
		Grand Total	

Add for shipping:
Book Rate: $2.50 for first item, $1.00 for ea. add. item.
First Class/UPS: $4.00 for first item, $1.50 ea. add. item.
Canada/Mexico: One-and-a-half times shipping rates.
Overseas: Double shipping rates.

Check type of payment:

☐ Check or money order enclosed

☐ Visa ☐ MasterCard

Acct. # ______________________

Exp. Date ______________________

Signature ______________________

Send order to:
Aslan Publishing
PO Box 108
Lower Lake, CA 95457
or call to order:
(800) 275-2606

NDLA